Help Your Dog Fight Cancer

D0208704

Help Your Dog Fight Cancer

Empowerment for Dog Owners

Turn Despair into Confidence
Become Your Best Friend's
Best Advocate

3rd edition

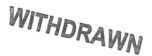

Laurie Kaplan
    Founder and Administrator of the Magic Bullet Fund
Alice Villalobos, DVM, Consultant
    Director, Animal Oncology Consultation Service, Hermosa Beach CA

This book is intended to educate owners of dogs with cancer to become better advocates for their dogs, communicate better with their veterinary medical team, and make better decisions for the benefit of their dogs.

The information in this book applies only to canines with cancer. Some of the therapies, treatments and methods discussed in this book may be harmful to pets of other species with or without cancer.

This book is not intended to replace veterinary medical advice or recommendations. Great care has been taken by the author to ensure the accuracy of information presented in this book. However, treatments, protocols or remedies described may not be suitable for your particular dog. Each dog's anatomy, condition, age, and medical history is unique and not all recommendations are appropriate for every dog. Author and publisher make no warranty, express or implied, regarding the efficacy of treatments or home care techniques discussed in this book and may not be held liable for consequences from treatments or techniques explicitly or implicitly described.

Appendix pages may be reproduced for distribution. No other pages in the book may be reproduced by any method for distribution to any person other than the purchaser without prior written permission of the publisher. No other pages may be posted anywhere on the Internet. Send requests for permissions to email@JanGenPress.com or call 914-941-0159. Books and eBooks can be ordered at www.jangenpress.com. Quantity discounts and clinic discounts available at site above, or call 914-941-0159.

3rd edition © 2016 Publisher JanGen Press
Library of Congress Control Number: 2015919134
ISBN: 978-0-9754794-3-8

2nd edition © 2008 Publisher JanGen Press
Library of Congress Control Number: 2008923705
ISBN: 978097547947-6

1st edition © 2004 Publisher JanGen Press
Library of Congress Control Number: 2004107152
ISBN: 0-9754794-6-6

Cover photograph by Tracy M. Basile

Table of Contents

This book is dedicated to Bullet,

the love of my life, the dog of my dreams,

my brave little boy,

and to all of the Brave Spirits who fight

for another shining moment

in the loving arms of their special person.

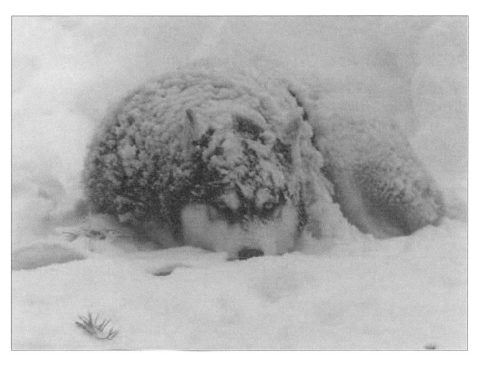

The Magic Bullet

March 15, 1991 ~ November 20, 2004

Foreword

by Bruce N. Hoskins, DVM

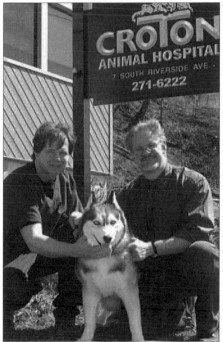

As a veterinarian in companion animal practice for more than twenty years, I have encountered many challenging cases and I have experienced, alongside my clients, many difficult losses. To me, however, the most difficult task I have to perform is that of informing a client their beloved pet has a disease that may prematurely end the pet's life.

Anyone fortunate enough to have experienced the unconditional love of a pet understands the mutual devotion that this relationship can foster and the profound sadness and distress that comes with news of a terminal illness. When the diagnosis is cancer, I see an added element of stress, stemming

Vet Tech Ed Mowan, Bullet, Dr. Hoskins

from the fear and frustration of dealing with the unknown.

Most of us have been touched by human cancer. We knew people who succumbed to the disease or to treatment, and we know people who are surviving. In contrast, most of my clients whose pets have cancer do not have a personal resource for information and support. Most do not have a friend who has seen their dog through cancer treatment. Through this book, Laurie has become that friend to many people.

I treated Bullet for many conditions for twelve years, ranging from the basic annual exam to Lyme Disease, bite wounds from altercations with other dogs and bone chips in his shoulder joint. He was a good patient, aside from the growls and complaints typical of the breed. Laurie was very much the devoted "mother," seeing Bullet through those spectacles of adoration that we all wear when we look at our pets. Still, she always responded to treatment recommendations with thoughtful consideration and objectivity. These are important elements for the caretaker of a canine cancer patient to develop in order to become an effective advocate.

Some clients are reluctant to ask questions, and become passive observers of their pet's cancer treatment. The author of this book is decidedly not in that client group. Laurie asked all of the questions that I expect a client might ask, and then went on to ask more.

Laurie was a true advocate for Bullet in every sense of the word. She went to great lengths to educate herself about Bullet's diagnosis, treatment and home-care options and potential complications. She challenged every member of Bullet's cancer team to research the hard questions and "think outside the box" to find solutions for Bullet.

I have been changed by my experience with Bullet and Laurie, especially during the four-plus years since Bullet's cancer diagnosis. He was my first patient to beat the odds and become a canine lymphoma survivor. Laurie never once lost faith in Bullet's ability to overcome cancer and, on more than one occasion, to survive severe treatment side effects and secondary complications. Through my relationship with Bullet and Laurie, I acquired a new respect for the power of a positive outlook and a team approach to the cancer fight, centered on the active involvement of the caretaker.

Veterinarians have written texts about canine cancer to be read by veterinarians. A few have written books for caretakers. Notably missing was a book written by a caretaker, for caretakers. In *Help Your Dog Fight Cancer*, Laurie offers such a book, full of information and support, to empower caretakers to become their dog's advocate and an active member of the team.

In July of 2000 I had the task of delivering a diagnosis of multicentric lymphoma in Bullet. It was a sad day, but it was the beginning of what was to become a poignant success story of canine cancer survival.

In November of 2004, Bullet died, never having come out of remission from lymphoma. I am happy to have been part of Bullet's cancer team. I am happy that I had the opportunity to work with Bullet, his cancer team, and his devoted human companion, Laurie Kaplan.

Thanks to You!

My Siberian Husky Bullet, the inspiration for this book, received excellent care before, during, and after his fight against cancer. I thank our primary care veterinarian, Dr. Bruce Hoskins, and the Croton Animal Hospital staff, for keeping Bullet healthy and strong throughout his life and for being ever tolerant of Bullet's antics (and mine).

Bullet received excellent care before, during, and after his fight against cancer. I thank our primary care veterinarian, Dr. Bruce Hoskins, and the Croton Animal Hospital staff, for keeping Bullet healthy and strong throughout his life, and for being ever tolerant of Bullet's antics (and my own).

The expertise of Bullet's cancer team is self-evident in Bullet's long survival. Dr. Paolo Porzio provided chemotherapy, and veterinary oncologist Dr. David Ruslander was our consultant. Both veterinarians provided invaluable guidance and support during Bullet's treatment and for the remainder of his life. A special thanks goes to Dr. Porzio for his tender loving care of Bullet in the clinic and on our long hikes, for the emotional support he provided me, and for convincing me to write the first edition of this book.

I thank Drs. Bea Ehrsam, Tina Aiken, and Marty Goldstein for Bullet's holistic care, and I thank Dr. Chris Angiello and the staff at the Katonah-Bedford Veterinary Center, in Bedford Hills, NY, for top-notch emergency care.

I thank all of the veterinary oncologists and veterinarians who took the time to provide me, via phone or email, with cutting-edge information for this book, including Drs. Phillip Bergman, Joe Impellizeri, Susan Cotter, Noel Berger, and W. Jean Dodds.

One year after Bullet's diagnosis, I discovered an online support group at Delphi Forums called Pet Cancer Support (PCS). PCS is a place to exchange information and emotional support for those who have a pet with cancer. This support is crucial to so many, especially to those who are alone in their battle and don't find support from friends and family. Thank you, Nancy Flom, for founding PCS and to all of the members in the early 2000s, too many to name, for showing me that I was not alone in my determination to fight canine cancer.

I thank all of the veterinary oncologists and veterinarians who have provided treatment for the dogs in the Magic Bullet Fund. Their recommendations and provision of supporting studies for treatment options helped me stay up to date on developments in canine cancer treatment.

A special thank you goes to Alice Villalobos, DVM, DPNAP. Dr. Villalobos is Director of Animal Oncology Consultation Service & Pawspice™ in Hermosa Beach California, was the 2005-2006 President of the American Association of Human Animal Bond Veterinarians, and was a recipient of the Leo Bustad Companion Animal Veterinarian Award for her role in bringing oncology services to companion animal practice.

In 2004, Dr. Villalobos recruited me to help her author a book about pet cancer. The result of our joint effort was a very helpful and successful text for veterinary school students and a reference for veterinarians providing cancer treatments to pets, titled: *Canine and Feline Geriatric Oncology: Honoring the Human-Animal Bond*.

Dr. Alice is the consultant for this book. For three years, Dr. Alice has provided answers to my many questions for clarification of the finer points of canine cancer treatment, and has provided a review of the entire content of this third edition of *Help Your Dog Fight Cancer*.

I have to thank all of the families in the Magic Bullet Fund for sharing with me their preferences, fears, and goals, and for allowing me to guide them in difficult decisions that must be made to help a dog fight cancer.

I thank the veterinarians who treated all of the dogs in the fund, many of whom discussed with me in depth the dog they were treating, to explore options and alternative treatments when treatment failed.

Last but not least, I thank you, the reader. I cringe with every new book order: "*Another dog has cancer.*" Nonetheless, I am happy that another dog and his loving owner will benefit from Bullet's experience and from the journey that Bullet and I took through canine cancer. Another person will keep Bullet's memory alive. The production of *Help Your Dog Fight Cancer* was a labor of love for Bullet, and for your dog as well.

Preface

About half of our dogs will have cancer in their lifetimes, yet most dog owners know little or nothing about caring for a dog with cancer. Not long ago, admittedly, there wasn't much to know. Today, however, treatment for canine cancer is nearly on par with treatment for human cancer, and there is a great deal to know.

If your dog has cancer, you're undoubtedly asking, *"What can I do?"* First, you will decide on a medical plan and put it into action. There are many considerations to take into account when choosing a plan, such as which diagnostic tests to allow, which veterinarian(s) to enlist, and which treatment you want your dog to have. There are almost always several treatments available, even when a veterinarian presents only one. This book will help you obtain information you were not given, and help you make the important decisions.

After you decide on a medical plan, you'll ask, *"What else can I do?"* The answer is, *Lots!* Regardless of what type of medical treatment you decide your dog should have (chemotherapy, radiation, surgery, an alternative therapy, or no treatment at all), there is a great deal more that you can do. You'll manage symptoms and side effects, and revise the treatment plan if necessary. You'll strengthen your dog's organs, and bolster his immune system. You'll help your dog better fight the disease and better tolerate the treatment, to improve his odds for survival.

When Bullet was diagnosed with lymphoma, I wanted to know what typically happens before, during, and after canine cancer treatment, and what else might happen that is not typical. I wanted to know what I should, shouldn't, could, and might do to help my dog survive. I wanted to know all of this right away, in plain English and without any. I wanted what you are reading right now. I wanted this book!

My experience as an animal writer and medical editor enabled me to delve into volumes of medical literature undaunted by medical lingo. My

1

mission was to become the best advocate I could for Bullet. I also consulted with general practice veterinarians, veterinary oncologists, holistic vets, oncologists in human medicine, and other owners of dogs with cancer. I researched treatment options, pharmaceuticals, supplements, nutraceuticals, diets, alternative treatments, and clinical trials. To find Bullet's home care regimen, I experimented extensively to find out what worked best.

What I discovered was that the more information I gathered and the more I understood about Bullet's condition, the more capable I felt of caring for him properly, and the more my anxiety diminished. This was my path to becoming the best advocate for my best friend. Now, I will help you become the best advocate for your dog. As you read, and your knowledge about canine cancer grows, your anxiety will wane. You will become a confident and competent advocate for your dog.

Paolo Porzio, DVM, who administered Bullet's chemotherapy, urged me repeatedly to write a book that would help other owners of dogs with cancer become knowledgeable and confident advocates. After a year, I resigned my position as editor of *Catnip*, a publication of Tufts University School of Veterinary Medicine, and set about writing the first edition of this book.

The information in this book was culled from reliable sources, including peer-reviewed veterinary publications and journals, veterinary oncologists, and veterinary school web sites, or is based on my own experiences helping Bullet and more than 400 Magic Bullet Fund dogs fight cancer. Through the Fund and in private consultations, I have helped hundreds of owners begin the bittersweet journey of living with and caring for a dog with cancer.

I launched the Magic Bullet Fund in conjunction with the publication of the first edition of this book, in 2004. I founded the Fund to offer financial assistance to people who have a dog with cancer but cannot afford treatment fees. As of October 2015, the Fund has helped more than 400 families provide cancer treatment for their dogs.

For many families, treatment is available but the costs are prohibitive. How terrible it must be to know that your dog would have a chance to survive if only you could afford treatment. Cancer survival may be a miracle, but for the families in the Magic Bullet Fund, just being able to see their dogs receive treatment is the real miracle. You can see the dogs and their families at www.themagicbulletfund.org.

All owners are initially overwhelmed, as was I, by the shocking news that their dog has cancer and by the prospect of losing their best friend. There are numerous ways to care for a dog with cancer. Each owner must choose the options that work best for the dog and the family.

This book will provide you with a solid foundation for your battle against canine cancer. You will come away from *Help Your Dog Fight Cancer* with confidence, prepared to begin the journey and to make informed decisions as your best friend's best advocate.

Cancer is a fierce enemy. To fight the good fight, we need all the ammunition we can get. Armed with information and love, you will discover the best possible way to care for your dog through the battle against cancer.

About Canine Cancer

People often ask me if the incidence of cancer in dogs is on the rise. It does seem to be on the rise, doesn't it? Just a few years ago, it was unusual to find a mention of dogs with cancer in any type of media. It was simply not an issue that held interest for the general public.

Now, there are many articles about canine cancer on local TV news channels, in newspapers and magazines. We see human interest stories about people helping their dogs fight cancer, about new treatments for dogs with cancer in development for human use, about veterinary oncologists and human oncologists collaborating to improve cancer treatments. We see wonderful success stories of dogs surviving cancer and inspirational stories of love and determination that owners express in their efforts to save their dogs' lives.

Everyone I speak to tells me about their dog with cancer, a friend's dog with cancer, a dog they read about with cancer, a dog who is in treatment and surviving cancer, or a dog who lost the battle against cancer.

At first I took it personally. I thought that I was reading and hearing about dogs with cancer at every turn simply because I write about dogs and cancer and I run a fund to help dogs with cancer. But no, there is more to it than that. It is not a figment of my imagination or selective hearing.

The Humane Society of the United States reported in 2013 that there are more than eighty-three million pet dogs in the United States. About half of them will develop some type of cancer during their lifetimes. This includes all types of malignancies, from small, incidental tumors that are easily removed, to terminal cancers. Here are a few interesting and sometimes conflicting statistics about a dog's risk for cancer.

The American Veterinary Medical Association (AVMA) reports that half of our dogs ten years or older will die because of cancer. The Animal Cancer Institute reports that about four million dogs are diagnosed with cancer each year. This translates to more than 16,000 a day. The National

Cancer Institute reports that about six million dogs in the United States are diagnosed with cancer each year, and that a dog is diagnosed with cancer every five seconds in the United States.. The Morris Animal Foundation reports that one in four dogs dies because of cancer. The Veterinary Oncology & Hematology Center in Norwalk, CT, reports that cancer is the number one natural cause of death in older cats and dogs, accounting for nearly 50 percent of pet deaths each year. And the ASPCA reports that 60 percent of all dogs over age six will have some kind of cancer in their lives.

As you can see, there are enough canine cancer statistics to make you dizzy. Making use of long-ago learned math skills (they said it would pay off someday) and my little calculator, I waded through the various statistics to discover this very conservative estimate:

Every day, 10,000 dogs in the U.S. are diagnosed with cancer.

It is difficult to determine whether or not there has been an increase in canine cancer. There was no such thing as a "veterinary oncologist" before about 1990. Board certification for veterinary oncology did not exist. Schools of veterinary medicine did not offer it.

Board-certified surgeons (or any veterinarian) could remove tumors, and generally that was the extent of treatment offered for pets with cancer. Chemotherapy, radiation therapy, and advanced surgery were not available. Those who had a dog with cancer other than a tumor that could be surgically removed were told to provide palliative care and prepare for the loss of their pet.

Cancer cases were not reported or catalogued or given a great deal of attention. Even today, with a plethora of canine cancer treatments going on, little reporting exists. Several agencies are attempting to create a database of pet cancers or a tumor database, but to my knowledge none are receiving the input they need from veterinarians to maintain a reference that is even close to being comprehensive.

There were a handful of pioneer veterinarians who specialized in cancer treatment for cats and dogs, offering treatments beyond tumor removal, but they were few and far between. One such pioneer is Dr. Alice Villalobos, DVM, in Hermosa Beach, California. Dr. Villalobos completed a first generation oncology residency program while earning her doctorate at UC Davis under the mentorship of Dr. Gordon Theilen, the forefather of veterinary oncology. Dr. Villalobos has been providing cancer treatment for her patients for more than forty years, long before the first "veterinary oncologist" received board certification.

Since 1990, the production of several generations of veterinary oncologists and the availability of cancer treatment for pets has led to an explosion in the diagnosis and treatment of pets with cancer. This may give the impression of, but should not be confused with, an increase in the actual incidence of pet cancer.

More than 10,000 dogs are diagnosed with cancer every day, but there are only about 250 veterinary oncology specialists in practice in the United States, holding board certification in veterinary oncology and trained to treat pets with cancer. This disparity in supply and demand has created an unparalleled boon in veterinary medicine not only for the board-certified cancer specialists, but also for many general practice veterinarians.

Because there are not enough board-certified oncologists to handle *all* of the cases, many general practice and internal medicine veterinarians have expanded and altered their practices to offer chemotherapy. Any veterinary clinic that provides chemotherapy can count on a plethora of new clients willing to go to great lengths to help their dogs survive.

Now that veterinary medicine offers advanced diagnostic and treatment options, owners of pets with treatable cases can take advantage of these tools and fight for a cure or a remission. Our willingness and determination to help our pets survive at any cost has changed the face of veterinary medicine.

Pet owners and veterinarians are not the only ones to benefit. The supplement market is flooded with products that claim to help pets fight cancer. For the supplement manufacturers, the spotlight on canine cancer is an opportunity to market their products to owners of pets with cancer. In some cases, the same products that have been on the market for many years are re-labeled and marketed for pets with cancer. The products may or may not actually help in the fight against cancer, for people or for pets.

According to a report in the third edition of *Pet Supplements and Nutraceutical Treats in the U.S.*, published by Packaged Facts in Feb 2011, pet supplement sales "are expected to reach $1.6 billion by 2015, a 27 percent increase from 2010."

Is there a higher incidence of cancer in pets? Until the 1990s, most pets with cancer were given a grim prognosis and owners were given information about palliative care and euthanasia. Since the 1990s, the availability of medical options for pets with cancer led to a marked increase in the number of pets *diagnosed with and treated for* cancer, but this doesn't necessarily mean that more pets are *developing* cancer.

Causes and Prevention

When a dog is diagnosed with cancer, many owners feel the weight of responsibility. They wonder, *Am I to blame? Did I expose my pet to something that caused this cancer? Did I neglect to provide something that would have protected my dog against cancer?* Don't waste your energy blaming yourself for your dog's cancer. It's impossible to completely protect a dog against this disease.

Cancer can develop in a dog even when the owner has provided perfect care. We don't know how to stop cancer from developing. All we can do is be careful to avoid known causes, be watchful for the warning signs and be prepared to act if cancer does arise.

Carcinogenic or Toxic Chemicals

Products that contain chemicals but are deemed safe for use by humans can harm, kill, or cause cancer in a dog. When we spray or sprinkle a product, the mist floats in the air and then some of it is carried to the ground by gravity. The fumes and residues may not harm us, but we're not inhaling them in a concentrated form. Once on the ground, they contact only the soles of our shoes.

But a canine's nose and mouth are close to the ground. Dogs sniff and lick anything that has an interesting odor. Our pets inhale or ingest so many particulates left over from the sprays and powders we use, that we might just as well add them to the food bowl!

The word "non-toxic" on a product label does not necessarily mean it's safe for a dog to breathe, lick off the floor, or lick off of his paws. For more information on toxins, contact the ASPCA Animal Poison Control Center at (888) 426-4435, or online at www.aspca.org/pet-care/poison-control.

Lawn care products may be the worst offenders. Find non-toxic lawn products, or use a garden flamer to burn away your weeds. Fertilizers, weed killers, and pesticides cause canine lymphoma. A 2003 study at Purdue University School of Veterinary Medicine concluded that they cause transitional cell carcinoma (TCC) in Scottish Terriers. This study showed that the risk of TCC significantly increased for the dogs exposed to lawns treated with herbicides and insecticides or herbicides alone.

Manufacturers of many lawn care products recommend that pets are kept off of the lawn for twenty-four hours after application. This may not be a strong enough warning to protect our dogs. The chemicals may be safe for us, but we don't roll around on the ground and dig in the dirt. We don't inhale the powders with our noses an inch from the ground.

Chemicals picked up outdoors on the soles of our shoes or our bare feet don't end up in our mouths. We don't lick the bottoms of our shoes or feet. But I know that Bullet did and, most likely, your dog does too.

Even if you're careful, a breeze or a leaf blower can carry the products your neighbors use on their lawns onto your yard. Despite all of your precautions, your dog may wind up licking those harmful chemicals off of his feet unless you have the authority to ban the use of chemical-laden lawn care products in your neighborhood.

Most of the pesticides that we spray on our bodies—including some natural ones and organic and non-toxic formulas—are labeled "not for internal use." If you use bug spray on your arm and your dog licks it, he is "using it internally."

We are a chemical-happy society. Many chemicals we use are entirely unnecessary. Get your kitchen floor squeaky clean by using hot water and a mild, natural soap. Clean any stubborn dirt remaining with an abrasive pad or a stronger cleanser. You will need more aggressive cleaning methods if you re-shoe horses or hose down competitors of a mud-wrestling match in your kitchen, but in most households cleansing with hot water and a mild cleanser is sufficient.

Many of the floor-polishing, carpet-cleaning, and oven-cleaning products that line the shelf in your supermarket contain chemicals that can cause cancer (carcinogens), if ingested. Most of the house-cleaning products in your health food store contain ingredients that are non-toxic but still unsafe to ingest.

9

Rinse and re-rinse your floors thoroughly after using any cleanser that you would not drink. If your dog is eating and a bit of food falls onto the floor, he will probably knock over the food and water bowl frantically, to get at that morsel, and lick the floor in the process.

You can make your own safe, non-toxic house cleaning solutions for just about any task. Certified herbalist Ernestina Parziale offers detailed instructions at earthnotes.tripod.com, on the "Cleaning Recipes" page.

More great tips for non-toxic house cleaning can be found here: http://eartheasy.com/green-home, and in a book by Karyn Siegel-Maier titled *The Naturally Clean Home: 150 Super-Easy Herbal Formulas for Green Cleaning* (Storey Publishing, LLC, December 1, 2008).

Cancer and Spayed, Neutered, or Intact Dogs

Many pet-related organizations work to educate the pet-owning public about spay/neuter as the solution to pet overpopulation. Millions of cats and dogs are euthanized each year simply because there aren't enough homes for them. After years of public outreach, many owners are now finally opting to spay or neuter their pets.

For those who don't find over-population a compelling enough reason to spay or neuter, there may be a more personal reason. Spay/neuter may be a way to significantly minimize a pet's risk for cancer of the reproductive organs. Ovarian cancer in females, and testicular cancer in males, can develop only if the reproductive organs are present. No ovaries means no ovarian cancer, and in most cases, no mammary cancer. No testicles means no testicular cancer.

Once a dog has cancer, should she be spayed or should he be neutered? Tony Henderson, in North Myrtle Beach, SC, was a dog helped by the Magic Bullet Fund. Tony had a mast cell tumor in his ear. He was eight years old and had not been neutered.

I spoke about this to Tony's veterinarian, Dr. Noel Berger, DVM, MS, Diplomate, American Board of Laser Surgery, at the Animal Hospital and Laser Center of South Carolina in Pawleys Island, SC. Dr. Berger offered the following explanation of why Tony should not be neutered:

"Tony is nine years old, well behaved, non-roaming, non-marking, non-aggressive and his old balls are not going to get anyone pregnant. As a

twenty-four year seasoned veteran practitioner, I understand the importance of spaying and neutering everything in sight, and I completely agree with your provisional requirement to have every candidate spayed or neutered. It sends a strong message to the general pet owning public, I get it.

For Tony, however, I strongly believe it is medically contraindicated to neuter him while he is having surgery and chemotherapy. He needs a source of endogenous testosterone to help him heal from surgery and defeat the cancer. Additionally, without his testosterone, the Vinblastine treatments may be much less effective.

Vinblastine enters the cells through a Calcium channel, mediated by sex hormone receptors. With sex hormones circulating, the channel can stay open longer, allowing more of the drug to cross into the cell membrane. It is the same story in males or females.

*It is not always this simple. Most of the time with female dogs, especially mammary cancer or vaginal masses, they **must** be spayed in order for chemotherapy to work. The drug taxolol, for example, works best in the absence of sex hormones, and the pet must be spayed or neutered for optimal effect."*

Until recently, the recommendation has been to spay/neuter dogs at a young age. New research shows that in some situations, a spayed or neutered pet may actually be at higher risk for some types of cancer.

A 2013 study at UC Davis provided interesting information. The study, titled, "Neutering Dogs: Effects on Joint Disorders and Cancers in Golden Retrievers," states that 759 Goldens were used and the results show that the intact dogs (male and female) had a significantly lower incidence of lymphoma, hemangiosarcoma and mast cell cancer.

Are Goldens representative of all dog breeds? A 2011 study titled "Long-term health effects of neutering dogs: comparison of Labrador Retrievers with Golden Retrievers," was published online by PLOS (Public Library of Science). The results of this study showed that in male and female Labrador Retrievers, spay/neuter at any age did not significantly effect the incidence of cancer. The study proposes that Goldens may be uniquely predisposed to develop cancer if spayed/neutered, in the absence of certain hormones.

What about mammary cancer? There is a study published in the *Journal of Small Animal Practice*, May 2012, titled "The Effect of Neutering on the Risk of Mammary Tumours in Dogs—a Systematic Review." This review suggests that there is no strong or sound evidence in the studies showing that spay/neuter can lower a pet's risk for cancer risk. It concludes that the studies are not a good basis for recommendations to spay and neuter.

Skin Cancer from the Sun

Harmful rays from the sun can cause skin cancer in dogs, including squamous cell carcinomas and hemangiomas. While all dogs are susceptible to cancers that develop because of exposure to the sun, the dogs at highest risk are those with a sparse coat, especially those with white or light-colored hair. A dog's underside, where the hair is sparse, and the face are most vulnerable areas, but legs and any part of the body can also be vulnerable if exposed to the sun's rays.

If your dog is at risk for skin cancer, apply protective cream when he is in the sun. Most creams for humans are not edible. You could use off-the-shelf SPF cream and instruct your dog not to lick it, but he probably will not obey. Look for a cream specifically for dogs, with a high sun protective factor (SPF).

In 1997, Bullet had double shoulder surgery for bone chips that may have resulted from our sledding outings. I knew this surgery was done arthroscopically for people, and I made an extra effort to find a surgeon who could perform the surgery arthroscopically. I wanted to make Bullet's recovery easier and the healing faster and avoid the extensive shaving necessary for open surgery.

When I picked Bullet up, he was shaved from ankle to neck on both sides and across the back. I was furious with the hospital and have not been there since. Over the next few days, Bullet's shaved skin turned all shades of black and blue, purple and yellow. Our general practice vet said it looked as though the surgical team used a razor with blades that weren't sharp.

It was a hot, sunny summer, and in 1997 there was no SPF cream yet available for dogs. I found a lip salve with SPF sun block and thought the manufacturer must realize that some of the product would

*get into our mouths and be ingested. I called the manufacturer and
learned that the cream was indeed safe to ingest. It took a long time
for Bullet's fur to grow in, and until it did, I used the lip salve on his
skin when we were outdoors for an extended period of time.*

Vaccinations

A link between a pet's vaccinations and the onset of cancer has been
suspected for many years. Many studies have been done attempting to
discover the reason for this link. None have succeeded. Vaccine-associated
sarcomas often develop at an injection site when vaccines are given repeatedly at the same place on a dog's body. These are more common in cats.

There is some evidence that the adjuvants in a vaccine, which give it a
longer shelf life, may lead to cancer. Using the longer-acting vaccines, such
as the three-year Rabies vaccine, can minimize the amount of adjuvant
given to a pet over its lifetime and the number of times a vaccine (with
adjuvants) is given to the pet.

In April 2001, AVMA issued the following statement. "*... some vaccines
provide immunity beyond one year. Revaccination of patients with sufficient
immunity does not add measurably to their disease resistance, and may increase
their risk of adverse post-vaccination events.*"

Veterinarians who still promote annual vaccinations remind us of
epidemics that have been avoided or curtailed and the thousands of dogs'
lives that have been spared by the vaccine. They vaccinate their own pets.
It doesn't make sense, they say, to risk losing a dog to a disease when there
is a vaccine available that can virtually guarantee to protect him from it.

For holistic and some traditional veterinarians, the annual vaccine
philosophy has fallen out of favor. Knowing that most vaccines are effective longer than one year, we can titer-test instead of vaccinating annually.
A titer test shows the protection level still in your dog's blood from past
vaccines. You can choose to vaccinate only for diseases and illnesses that
are truly a threat in your region, and only when the previous vaccine is no
longer present in your dog's blood at an effective level.

In general, dogs with cancer who are not aggressive should not be
vaccinated. The Rabies Vaccine is required by most states, but a waiver can
be requested for a dog with cancer. Read more about vaccines and cancer
in the "Whole Health" chapter.

13

Genetics

Genetics play a role in a dog's risk for cancer. Cancer is more likely to arise in some dog breeds than others. A particular breed may be predisposed to develop cancer in general or a specific type of cancer. A predisposition to cancer can be due to unfortunate genetic defects or mutations, which can be perpetuated through breeding.

In other cases, cancer develops not because of a genetic mutation but because of the genetically determined definition of the breed. For example, large and giant breed dogs are more likely to develop osteosarcoma. A twenty-pound dog and a one hundred and fifty-pound dog will both reach their full size in approximately two years. However, one dog's leg bone must grow from two inches long to six inches long in the same period of time that it takes another dog's leg bone to grow from two inches long to twenty-four inches long. The accelerated growth that is necessary may be the explanation for a higher incidence of bone cancer that is seen in large and giant breed dogs.

Responsible breeders follow up on their progeny and keep medical records for the dogs they have sold. Without such follow-up, breeders may continue to mate a pair that repeatedly produces pups with cancer. Breeders should be aware when cancer develops in a breeding line and stop breeding the pair.

Apoptosis is a natural cellular mechanism that causes cells to die a natural death. Healthy cells are programmed for apoptosis. Genetic mutations, whether inborn or acquired, can disable the apoptosis process by making the cells incapable of natural cell death. As a result, the cells do not expire as they should. This interruption in cellular function is a contributing factor in most if not all cancers.

Diet and Cancer

What does your dog eat? The quality of meat used in pet foods should be scrutinized. Commercial dog food has been found to contain sick or downed cows and even meat from dead dogs.

Fruits, vegetables, and grains may contain pesticides, dyes, and bleach. Genetically modified products aren't well labeled, and long-term effects of GMO foods are unknown. In *Food Pets Die For*, by Ann N. Martin (New Sage Press, 2003), the author writes, "Many of the grains used in commercial pet food contain levels of herbicides, pesticides, and fungicides that are cancer-causing agents." Grains that don't pass inspection for use in human foods are often deemed adequate for use in pet foods.

In 2007, after a number of pet deaths and great number of sick pets, the chemical melamine was discovered in commercial pet foods, prompting a barrage of recalls by many different pet food manufacturers.

Pet owners have become educated and more selective about their dog food purchases. Many companies have changed their ways, and some horrifying practices have been abandoned. Now that pet care has become a multi-billion-dollar industry, a slew of "all natural," organic, and home ade dog foods are available for those who can afford the pricey products.

You may think that preparing your pet's food will be expensive. It can cost less than buying a medium-level mass-produced food. When choosing ingredients, select the meats and vegetables that happen to be on sale. Preparing your pet's food is not as time-consuming as you might think either. Can you spare two to four hours one Sunday a month to prepare a month's worth of food for your dog?

Preparing "Bullet's Cancer Diet" is an option! It will not cost more than what you are paying now, and it will take a small amount of your time. This diet is very flexible with a lot of room to improvise. (See Bullet's Cancer Diet.)

If you want to be sure your pet eats healthy food, make it yourself!

There is another important benefit to preparing your dog's food with your own hands and giving up a bit of your precious time to do it. Every time you serve a meal, you will feel a bond with your dog much deeper than what you feel when you scoop food into the bowl from a can or pour it from a bag. Your heart will be full because there are not only good ingredients in the bowl, but you are feeding your dog from your heart.

Canine obesity can cause bladder cancer. Feed your dog a healthy diet, and monitor his weight so that you can adjust the amount of food properly. If your dog is gaining weight, make his meals smaller. If he is losing weight, make his meals larger. Don't blindly follow the manufacturer's instructions for meal sizes. Each dog has a unique metabolism and different requirements for food amounts.

Do not give your dog food every time he approaches you with a whine or a play bow. When you are busy, it's easy to say, "Oh, he just wants food," but maybe he actually wants *you*! Give him some of your time instead of food. Take him for a walk, or throw a ball. You may be surprised when he curls up afterward, no longer nudging or whining. His hunger didn't disappear. His desire for your attention was satisfied.

Cancer Treatment can Cause Cancer

Surgery, chemotherapy, and radiation therapy are the tools used to fight cancer. It may seem logical that the stronger the treatment and the more treatment given, the better the chances of eradicating the cancer. This is not the case. While the treatment is working to stop the cancer, it also has the potential to cause cancer. Paradoxically, cancer treatment can increase the risk for cancer.

People often ask me if surgery can make the cancer stronger than ever. They have heard that when a tumor is subjected to surgery but is not entirely removed, or when the tissues are exposed to air, the cancer explodes into high gear.

There may be some truth to this. As a tumor develops, new blood vessels also develop to supply that tumor with blood. This is called angiogenesis. When a tumor is completely removed, its blood vessels shrivel and die because the tumor is no longer demanding a blood supply.

When a tumor is incompletely removed, its blood vessels could provide a source of blood to help the remnants of the tumor recover and grow. The postsurgical tumor mass is smaller and the blood supply is set up to support a larger mass, so the cancer may be able to take hold and progress more quickly.

As mentioned earlier, chemotherapy and radiation therapy can increase the risk for cancer. These treatments are designed to damage the DNA in the cancer cells. Damaged cells are always at risk for becoming cancer cells. While many cancer cells are damaged during chemo or radiation, some healthy cells are also damaged, putting them at risk for DNA mutations and cancer.

Giving more treatment than necessary puts a dog at risk for myelosuppression, neuropathy, extravasation and a myriad of other chemotherapy side effects. (See "Overtreatment, page 112.)

Early Detection

We know that early detection in humans greatly improves the chances of treatment success. The same is true for pets. All pet owners should be familiar with the early warning signs of cancer. When cats and dogs aren't feeling well, they often mask the signs. They just keep plugging along because they don't know that they should tell us that something is wrong and they don't know how. If you are not paying attention, you will miss the opportunity to fight an illness early, when you may be able to beat it.

The key to finding cancer early, to give your dog the best chance of survival, is to be very observant of his appearance and behavior.

Notice your dog's eating and drinking habits so you will be aware of any changes. When walking your dog, notice his posture, speed, gait, and attitude, and the color and solidity of his stools when he makes a pit stop.

Annual exams are important even if your dog does not get annual vaccines. If you do not give your pet vaccines, ask your veterinarian to do titer tests annually instead. Also allow your veterinarian to draw your dog's blood for a complete blood count (CBC) and chemistry panel, and to collect or extract urine for urinalysis. Your vet should check your dog's teeth and gums and feel his body for lumps and bumps. The old ballpark estimate that there are seven "dog years" to each human year means that a checkup once a year for your pet is comparable to a checkup once every seven years for you.

10 Early Warning Signs of Cancer (Provided by AVMA)
- Abnormal swellings that persist or continue to grow
- Sores that do not heal
- Weight loss
- Loss of appetite
- Bleeding or discharge from any body opening
- Offensive odor
- Difficulty eating or swallowing
- Hesitation to exercise or loss of stamina
- Persistent lameness or stiffness
- Difficulty breathing, urinating, or defecating

See the "Early Warning Signs" list in the Appendix of this book for a more comprehensive list of early warning signs to watch for.

At Home Checkups

Below is a list of important items to include in a monthly at home checkup, provided for this book by Dr. Rodney Page, DVM, DACVIM (internal medicine, oncology), director of Colorado State University's Animal Cancer Center after eleven years at Cornell University College of Veterinary Medicine. All dog owners should examine their dogs monthly. For a dog diagnosed with cancer, do the checkup, at least once a week.

> ▶ Feel your dog's lymph nodes. See the map of lymph node locations and/or ask your veterinarian to show you where the nodes are on your dog.
> ▶ Feel the mammary glands on female dogs to detect any changes.
> ▶ Carefully examine the skin of your dog's entire body. Make "dermal maps" of any existing lumps and bumps. This will later help you determine how quickly a benign skin bump may be changing.
> ▶ Try to examine the inside of your dog's mouth. If your dog is agreeable, look for any lumps, swellings, or discolorations in the gums, teeth, roof, and under the tongue. If your dog is not so agreeable, ask your vet to inspect this area at your appointments.
> ▶ Annual blood and urine tests are adequate unless there are any abnormalities. Schedule rechecks every four to six months to follow any abnormal results.
> ▶ In breeds that are genetically at risk for splenic hemangiosarcoma, such as Golden Retrievers, German shepherd dogs, and Portuguese water dogs, owners should have these tests done twice a year if possible, as well as chest x-rays(radiographs) and an abdominal ultrasound.

Enlarged lymph nodes are a very important early warning sign. They indicate that something is wrong—an illness, an infection, or cancer. In most cases, the first sign of canine lymphoma is swollen or enlarged lymph nodes.

Feel the nodes regularly, and make a note of their sizes in your journal. The size of a node can be described well in relation to a food. For example, a node may be comparable in size to a pea, grape, walnut, or lemon.

There is a matching right-and-left set for each of the five external nodes shown. This is helpful because if the right inguinal node, for example, is larger than the left, clearly it is enlarged. In most dogs, you won't be able to feel the nodes at all when they are inactive and not enlarged. Inform your veterinarian immediately if the nodes suddenly feel larger.

Lymph Node Locations

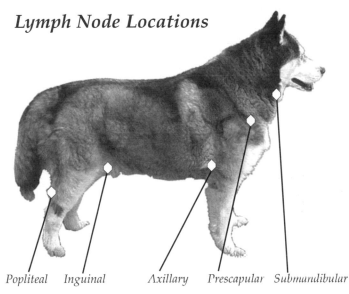

Popliteal   Inguinal   Axillary   Prescapular   Submandibular

Lymph node enlargement is often the first sign of cancer and the first sign of a relapse (out of remission). For each node shown, there is a matching node on the other side of the dog.

Cancer is not the only reason lymph nodes become enlarged, so don't panic! Take your dog to the veterinarian and he will determine the cause. Lymph nodes become enlarged when an infection is present. When your own doctor puts his hand around your throat during your annual checkup, he is feeling your submandibular lymph nodes to make sure they are not enlarged.

Whether your dog has cancer or not, give him regular at home check-ups. If you notice anything you don't expect, call your clinic. They will tell you whether you should have the vet examine your dog now or just mention it at your next appointment.

Our dogs can't speak up when they don't feel well. It's important to feel and watch and take note of their appearance, their behavior, and their habits. Illness can progress quickly, and the best chance of getting a good treatment result for any illness is to begin treatment as early as possible.

I was dreading the day Bullet would come out of remission. "How will I know? When might it be? What will happen next?" That feeling of being unprepared, of not knowing what to expect, was creating anxiety. The solution was to get some hard, cold facts, so I asked for some. Dr. Porzio said Bullet's lymph nodes would suddenly become enlarged. "Might I miss it?" I asked. "Like golf balls!" he said. He showed me where these golf balls would appear.

I began to check for lymph node enlargement every day. I would disguise the check as a petting and massaging session! I would scratch the top of his head, tweak his ears, run my fingers down his back along the spine ... and also check the locations where the nodes resided. I stopped the daily checks a year after Bullet's chemotherapy ended, but I continued to check them once in a while.

2

The Most Common Types of Canine Cancer

The list of cancers that appear in dogs is very similar to the list of cancers that are seen in people. Treatments available for a dog with cancer are also similar to the treatments used for humans with the same type of cancer. These facts are the basis for the rise of comparative oncology, and the use of our dogs to research for better treatments for human cancers.

Each type of cancer has a different prognosis, and different treatments that are effective. It is important to find out what type of cancer your dog has. Once you have that information, you can find out what treatments are used for the disease, compare survival rates and success rates and decide on a treatment plan.

After defining a type of cancer, there may also be sub-types as well as a stage and a grade that can all be discovered through diagnostic tests. In some cases, all of this information is irrelevant to the selection of a treatment plan. In other cases, the additional information is important.

When finances are tight, it may be possible to decide on a treatment plan regardless of sub-type, stage and grade. You can bypass the testing and simply provide the treatment that would be used for the sub-type that is most likely. If you are planning to provide aggressive treatment regardless of how aggressive or advanced the cancer is, testing for stage and grade is irrelevant. Just give the treatment.

After a surgery, you can have a biopsy done. This is always optional. If you already know that you are, or that you are not, going to proceed with treatment after the surgery, then the biopsy is irrelevant. If the surgery is the only treatment you plan on, then you can tell your veterinarian not to send the tissue to the lab, and not to include a fee for biopsy on your invoice. Even when the sub-type, stage and grade will not alter the treatment plan, you may still want to know all there is to know about your dog's cancer. If you can afford to, you can have all diagnostic tests done.

Tumors

The most common broad category of cancers in dogs are tumors that appear as lumps and bumps. They may be cutaneous (in the skin) or subcutaneous (under the skin). These tumors occur at a rate of 450 cases per 100,000 dogs per year. This means that approximately 274,000 dogs are diagnosed with skin cancer each year. Of these tumors, 70 to 80 percent are benign (such as lipomas).

When a dog has a benign tumor, the vet may recommend a "watch and wait" policy. If the tumor grows or bleeds or changes in any way, it should be tested and surgically removed if possible. If not removed, benign lipomas can undergo malignant transformation to become malignant liposarcomas.

When a dog has a mass on or in the skin, the vet may make a preliminary diagnosis from the appearance or feel of the lump. Unless your vet is sure that the lump is not malignant, ask for a fine-needle aspirate (FNA), Tru-Cut biopsy, or a surgical biopsy. For those who do not intend to give their dog additional treatment such as surgery, chemotherapy, or radiation therapy, there is no reason for any biopsy.

Mast Cell Cancer (Mastocytoma; MCT)

About 20 percent of cutaneous and subcutaneous tumors in dogs are MCTs, occurring at a rate of 129 per 100,000 dogs. Benign MCTs are called mastocytomas; malignant MCTs are called mastocytosarcomas. The following discusses treatment options for malignant MCT.

The prognosis is relatively optimistic when there is a single grade I or II tumor that can be surgically removed with clean margins. When possible, MCTs are surgically removed. Whether a dog has follow-up treatment or not, there may be no new tumors and no recurrent tumors for years. On the other hand, a new or recurring tumor may develop quickly *with or without* treatment. Choosing a treatment plan is difficult for this type of cancer, especially grade I or II, because of its unpredictable nature.

The prognosis worsens when the cancer has spread, or become systemic (metastatic), when there are multiple tumors in different locations, or when the grade is higher than grade II. In that case, your veterinarian will help you decide whether to give aggressive treatment or palliative care. Prednisone (a steroid) can be used for palliative care and may extend a dog's survival by a few months.

Depending on the size and location of the tumor, clean margins may not be obtainable during surgery. Then, it is certain that after surgery there are still cancer cells in the area. Without clean margins, or if the tumor is not operable at all, chemotherapy or radiation therapy will be recommended.

▷ *Manny Eno's Story*

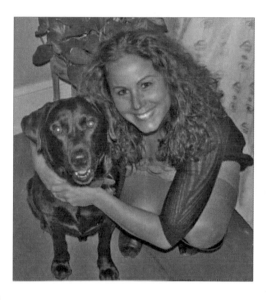

In early 2009, Manny had a lump in his groin area. Our vet Dr. Hirsch at West Roxbury Animal Hospital examined it and diagnosed a non-cancerous fatty tumor. He said if it changed in color or size, to bring Manny back for surgery.

Several months later, it did change. Manny had surgery and the biopsy results came back positive for grade II mast cell cancer.

At New England Veterinary Oncology Group, veterinary oncologist Dr. Philibert suggested that Manny should have another surgery to remove the tissue that surrounded the tumor. He explained that it's important to not only remove the tumor but to also remove the tissue that surrounded it, in case there were any cancerous cells left behind.

Manny had the second surgery. After his incision healed, they tested to determine if the cancer had spread to other areas of his body. The results showed no signs of the cancer spreading and Dr. Philibert said that now Manny should have twelve radiation treatments.

The whole radiation experience was surprisingly easy on Manny. He had no major side effects, just minor "sunburn" in his groin area.

*Manny was examined periodically for the first year to make sure the
cancer hadn't come back.*

*It's now almost four years since Manny was diagnosed with mast
cell cancer and he is happier and healthier than ever!*

- Kathryn Eno, Jamaica Plain, Massachusetts

Another option is follow-up treatment with one of the newly developed medications for mast cell cancer. These are tyrosine kinase inhibitors (TKIs). Products developed and in use so far include Palladia (toceranib), and Kinavet® or Masivet® (masitinib; AB1010). Masitinib is the active ingredient of the first-ever registered veterinary anticancer drug, Masivet. FDA description of Masitinib is that it was conditionally approved in 2010 "for treatment of recurrent (post-surgery) or non-resectable grade II or III cutaneous mast cell tumors in dogs that have not previously received radiotherapy and/or chemotherapy except corticosteroids."

Dogs may be given these drugs indefinitely, or until side effects arise. Periodic blood tests will be necessary to assess the efficacy of the drug. Drug dosages are often tapered off gradually.

Of the three, Palladia seems to have more side effects than either Masivet or Kinavet. Side effects generally are gastrointestinal. When they do arise, consult your veterinarian right away. Often a vet will recommend switching to one of the other tyrosine kinase inhibitors. When side effects are severe, you have the option to use a different treatment, or to stop treatment and provide palliative care.

When a biopsy report shows incomplete surgery and dirty margins, further treatment should be considered. This should not be confused with a biopsy report stating that clean margins were attained but "microscopic disease may remain." In that case, further treatment is not necessarily indicated. This verbiage is very effective at making the owner fearful that the cancer will return. To be more accurate and less terrifying, the report should state: "Microscopic disease may *or may not* remain."

▷ **Stella Festino's Story**

*I adopted Stella in 2007, at three years old. One year later, I felt
bumps under her chin. Our family veterinarian, Dr. Mary A.
Birmingham at Sayrebrook Veterinary Hospital, did a fine needle aspi-*

*rate and a few days later they called me
with the horrific news that Stella had
mast cell cancer.*

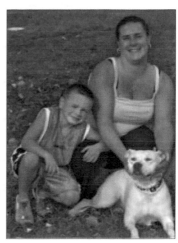

*We could not afford the medical
treatment she needed. We had just lost
our home to foreclosure and I had filed
for bankruptcy. In July 2008, the Magic
Bullet Fund paid for Stella's surgery.*

*The biopsy showed that it was grade
II mast cell cancer and recommended a
consult with a radiation oncologist. I did
not want Stella to have radiation treatments. I trusted that the surgery was
done properly and that she did not need further treatment.*

*That was six years ago. Since then, Stella has had two minor
surgeries to remove small lumps—one in December 2011 and another
in July 2013.*

*I am comfortable with my decision not to give Stella radiation. I
know that she could have developed these additional lumps even if
she did have the radiation treatments. I just check her whole little
body for lumps regularly and have them removed right away.*

*At ten years old, Stella is her happy, cheerful puppy self who loves
everyone. She was given another chance at life and many more
wonderful years with my family.*

- Jennifer Festino, Sayreville, New Jersey

Canine Malignant Melanoma (CMM)

Melanoma most often develops on darkly pigmented skin. CMM
tumors arise in the skin, orally, on a digit, or internally. About 6 percent of
all canine tumors are melanomas. Melanoma is a very aggressive cancer.

Historically, there has been no effective treatment for this deadly and
fast moving cancer, but a tyrosinase DNA vaccine called ONCEPT® was
approved recently, specifically for the treatment of oral CMM.

Dr. Phil Bergman, who developed the vaccine in conjunction with
oncologists at Sloan Kettering, told me that "Early results show that this
vaccine may double or triple survival time." ONCEPT®, from Merial, has

been approved by the FDA for veterinary use and is available as a vaccine. It is injected via a canine transdermal device once every two weeks for four treatments. A booster is given every six months.

According to Dr. Bergman, "The Xenogeneic DNA vaccination should be considered as an adjunctive therapy for CMM patients with minimal residual disease and/or low tumor burden." Xenogeneic means "from a different species." In this case, the tyrosinase that is injected into the dog is human tyrosinase. The vaccination induces an antibody response in dogs with advanced melanoma, and the increased antibodies are thought to attack CMM cancer cells.

However, a 2013 article titled "A Retrospective Analysis of the Efficacy of ONCEPT Vaccine for the Adjunct Treatment of Canine Oral Malignant Melanoma," was published in *Veterinary and Comparative Oncology*. The abstract of the article states that, "The purpose of this study was to determine whether adjunctive treatment with the ONCEPT melanoma vaccine affected the outcome of dogs with OMM [oral malignant melanoma] that had achieved loco-regional cancer control... Dogs that received the vaccine did not achieve a greater progression-free survival, disease-free interval or median survival time than dogs that did not receive the vaccine."

▷ *Ukiah Burton's Story*

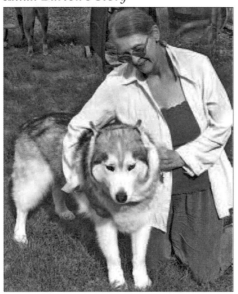

In March of 2008, Ukiah was dumped in my yard with heartworms, hookworms and pneumonia. His pads were bleeding and his fur was stinking and matted. He weighed less than sixty pounds. Our veterinarian, Dr. K. Reynolds at Clio Animal Hospital, estimated his age at about two and a half years old.

In March of 2010, during a routine dental cleaning, the vet found a two centimeter "spot" in Ukiah's mouth.

It was removed, but without clean margins, and diagnosed as oral melanoma. We were given hope and help by Laurie Kaplan. Thanks to the wonderful Magic Bullet Fund, Ukiah was started on his miraculous road to recovery. Ukiah had six radiation treatments by Dr. Amy M Koterbay at MSU Veterinary Oncology Teaching Hospital in Lansing, Michigan.

Ukiah is now is a member of a study that monitors his progress thru his DNA. His progress will help other dogs diagnosed with this form of cancer. He still receives the Merial DNA Vaccine every six months.

I remember the fear and sorrow I felt when I first heard Ukiah's diagnosis. I believed it was a death sentence. But he is still going strong and as of July 2014, Ukiah is a 52-month survivor of oral melanoma and he is still going strong!

- Pamela Burton, Flint, Michigan

There has been a flurry of research into new ways to treat canine cancer, and in large part it is because dogs serve as a very useful model for the development of human cancer treatments. Dogs respond to treatments much more quickly than do humans. Therefore, the success of a new treatment can be discovered more quickly when it is tested on dogs.

Despite the excitement of oncologists and veterinarians who are testing treatments on dogs toward development of human cancer treatments, there is a possible drawback. While it is true that treatments work (or don't work) more quickly in dogs, it is also true that the cancer spreads more quickly in dogs. It is possible that in some of the trials, test results are less useful than hoped for because the dogs die from cancer before they are able to complete the treatment being tested.

Dermal Hemangiosarcoma

Hemangiosarcoma tumors most often arise in the heart or the spleen, but can appear in or under the skin in lightly pigmented areas that are exposed to the sun. Is dermal, subcutaneous, or hypodermal hemangiosarcoma, the tumors are not highly malignant. These tumors should be surgically removed as soon as possible.

After surgery, dermal hemangiosarcoma provides a longer expected survival time than does cardiac or splenic hemangiosarcoma. If performed before metastasis has taken place, surgery can provide survival of two years without any follow-up treatment. In rare cases, early surgery may successfully remove the cancer entirely, and the dog may then live out his natural life.

Soft Tissue Sarcomas (STS)

Sarcomas are malignant tumors. About 15 percent of cutaneous and subcutaneous tumors in dogs are soft tissue sarcomas. They include liposarcoma, fibrosarcoma, peripheral nerve sheath tumor (schwannoma), histiocytoma, hemangiopericytoma, leiomyosarcoma, rhabdomyosarcoma, and hemangiosarcoma (see above).

Treatments and prognoses for this type of cancer vary according to the type of sarcoma. As a rule, these cancers are difficult to eradicate. The best course of action is complete tumor removal as early as possible, with wide and clean margins if possible. After complete tumor removal, the average survival is three and a half years. With surgery and radiation, average survival is six and one-quarter years. For an older dog, where a three-year survival would place the dog in geriatric years and a six-year survival would be unheard of, giving radiation might not make sense.

Fibrosarcomas are soft tissue sarcomas of the connective tissue. They arise in or under the skin anywhere on the body, or in the mouth. Oral fibrosarcomas are malignant and are destructive to local tissues. After surgical removal, these tumors may recur but slowly. Small tumors may not return for more than a year. Larger tumors (more than four centimeters) may return in less than a year. Oral fibrosarcoma does not tend to metastasize as quickly as oral melanoma does.

Carcinomas

The most common carcinomas are anal sac carcinoma, transitional cell carcinoma, and mammary carcinoma. For anal sac tumors, surgery is recommended to remove the primary tumor and possibly one or more lymph nodes if they are found to contain cancer cells. Surgery may be followed by chemotherapy with doxorubicin and Cytoxan, or doxorubicin and 5-fluorouracil. Anal sac tumors comprise two percent of all skin tumors in dogs.

▷ **Marley Thayer's Story**

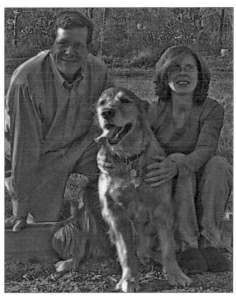

In September 2003, a good friend, breeder and fellow pet therapy member had a litter of puppies. My family (me, husband Tad, and our son and daughter) all went to meet the puppies, even though we had recently lost our dear Golden, Jorden, to cancer and we didn't think we were ready for another dog. But we met puppy Marley and we couldn't resist. We brought him home for my birthday in November.

If I say Marley was the best dog ever, I am not exaggerating. He was smart, beautiful, loving, and was a natural as a therapy dog. We took him to hospitals, schools and nursing homes. The loving nature of Goldens is why we have always been attracted to them.

In the summer of 2010, Marley had a seizure that lasted for a minute or so. When it happened again, we took him to our vet in Middletown, NY. Dr. Barra felt an enlargement on Marley's neck so he did diagnostic tests and found that Marley had a tumor on his thyroid. Dr. Barra explained that an artery going to his brain was being compressed by the tumor, hence the seizures. He removed the tumor in August 2010.

Dr. Barra said he couldn't be positive whether or not any cancer remained, so we saw veterinary oncologist Dr. Joe Impellizeri. After testing, he did not find any evidence that the cancer remained but he recommended that Marley have four to six chemotherapy treatments. We agreed because we couldn't stand thinking that there was something we could do to help Marley, and we were not doing it.

Dr. Impellizeri gave Marley four chemo treatments with Carboplatin, beginning in September of 2010 and ending in December. In the middle of the chemo treatment plan, we ran out of *money, but the Magic Bullet Fund helped us finish Marley's last three chemo treatments. I read Laurie's book [this book] and got Marley on the diet and supplements that would help him fight cancer.*

Marley was fine with a great quality of life for seven months. Then, in May 2011, Marley suddenly became weak and bloated. Our vet diagnosed kidney failure. We brought him home with medication and he died at home with us.

I later learned that Carboplatin can cause kidney damage. If I had it to do over, I would not put him through the chemo.

We haven't gotten another dog since we lost Marley. I love every-thing about Goldens except, of course, cancer. After having two in a row with cancer, we now know how susceptible they are to cancer. I do want another Golden and will do my best to find a breed line without cancer. I love their beauty, intelligence, personalities and I love other Golden owners.

Carol Thayer, Wappinger's Falls, New York

Transitional cell carcinoma (TCC) is the most common type of bladder cancer in dogs. The tumor begins in the bladder and spreads to the lymph nodes, liver, and lungs. When the tumor causes urethral obstruction, urination is blocked, and this is a life-threatening situation.

Surgical removal of the tumor is the best plan, but TCC tumors are often inoperable. A six-month survival is possible if the dog is given an NSAID such as piroxicam. This may be given with or without chemother-apy. The chemo drug usually given is Novantrone® (mitoxantrone). The average survival, regardless of treatment selection, is less than a year.

▷ **Cadence Montellano's Story**

In the summer of 2012, at ten years old, our sweet Cadence began to have trouble urinating. Our veterinarian found crystals in her urine, diagnosed bladder stones, and we changed her diet to a prescription dog food. One month later, we discovered that she had a tumor called transitional cell carcinoma on her bladder.

Our vet told us that the CSU Flint Animal Cancer Center in Fort Collins, Colorado, might be able to help. Cadence would be given intensity-modulated, image-guided radiation therapy every week-day with anesthesia, as well as chemotherapy treatments. The survival rate for dogs given this treatment is more than double any other treatment method.

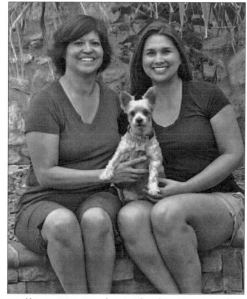

That was good news, but we still had no money! We didn't know what to do until some research brought us to the Magic Bullet Fund. The Fund donated part of Cadence's treatment cost and helped us raise the rest.

In September 2012, we drove twelve tense, worried hours from El Paso, TX to Fort Collins, CO. Cadence had to stay at the hospital there for a month. When the month was over, we picked up our baby. It was the best day ever! Although we were still worried, Dr. Susan LaRue said she didn't want to give us false hope, but "She got that cancer good"!

Cadence was very, very thin. She had lost a lot of weight. She also had radiation burns in her vaginal area, but they healed perfectly after about a month. The radiation had turned her naturally light colored skin and fur color dark. For the first two weeks home, Cadence was lethargic but she was so very happy to be home. It took a few more weeks for her to start feeling better, and then from that time forward she was such a happy baby!

At one year since Cadence was diagnosed, she was in good spirits, showing no sign that anything was ever wrong. She turned eleven and then twelve years old.

Cadence passed away on October 29, 2014. She lived more than two years after her cancer diagnosis. We were so fortunate to have our baby in our lives and to get to spend extra time with her. She is missed every single day and remembered with fond memories.

- Rachel G Montellano and Salina Cobos, El Paso, Texas

In May 2014, Dr. LaRue told me that she continues to treat patients with this protocol. Dr. LaRue says, "This week in the clinics we are retreating a dog who was treated three years ago. We have had some very impressive outcomes." (See *Journal of Veterinary Internal Medicine*, 2012 article titled "Intensity-Modulated and Image-Guided Radiation Therapy for Treatment of Genitourinary Carcinomas in Dogs.")

▷ **Molly Burton's Story**

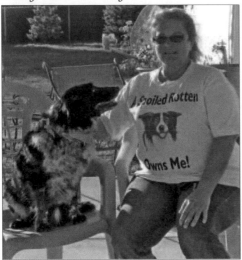

On March 11, 2010, our veterinarian glided the ultrasound probe over Molly's abdomen. There was silence, and then that word: Cancer. Molly had transitional cell carcinoma. The vet said surgery was not an option, due to the location of the tumor.

Oncologist Dr. Nancy Kay explained to us that the prognosis was poor, and that Molly would survive six to eighteen months. I was shocked and scared, but already my hackles were up and I was ready to fight. No time for a pity party!

Treatment started with Peroxicam and Mitoxantrone. Molly responded well and the tumor shrank. Five months later, treatment stopped working and the tumor began to grow. The chemo drug Carboplatin was not effective, but Vinblastine was. One year after her diagnosis, Molly had plenty of energy, and she was happy.

When you have a dog with bladder cancer, you become obsessed with their urine and urination habits. How much? How often? How fast? What color? Molly probably thought I'd lost my mind, but I found these observations to be invaluable.

August 2011, my vigilance paid off. Molly's tumor had grown thickly down her urethra and urination was nearly impossible. At UC Davis, Dr. William Culp placed a urethral stent and the urine flowed *in rivers! That stent saved Molly's life. One week later, Molly was joyfully doing a full Agility course of twelve obstacles.*

In January 2012, the tumor was occupying 90 percent of her bladder. Dr. Jakubiak in Concord, CA had come across a human protocol (Gemzar and docetaxel given on the same day with a few hours in between), which he had adapted for dogs with TCC. Oncologist Dr. Sita Withers agreed to use the protocol on Molly. Her ultrasound after three treatments showed no tumor growth.

In June, 2012 we tried one more chemo drug and Molly sailed through the first nine weeks, but then became ill. We agreed to stop chemotherapy. I continued acupuncture, supplements and antibiotics.

In February 2013, Molly's tumor started to bleed and we could not stop the bleeding. On February 26, 2013, two weeks shy of the three-year mark since diagnosis, I took Molly to UC Davis where the vets had fallen in love with her. Together, we decided it was time to let Molly go. She passed peacefully, surrounded by love, her eyes calmly glued to mine as if to say "Everything is going to be fine, Mom. Thank you."

Molly's quality of life throughout the journey was very good, playing Frisbee up until a few days before she left us. Would I go through the journey of fighting canine cancer again, with all of the ups and downs? Absolutely!

- Joellen & Mark Burton, Sebastopol, California

Cutaneous T-Cell Lymphoma (CTCL)

Lymphoma may be T-cell or B-cell. T-cell lymphoma is less common by far, and statistics vary greatly in veterinary literature, but human oncology reports that 16 percent of malignant lymphoma cases are T-cell. T-cell lymphoma requires different treatment from B-cell lymphoma, and the prognosis is not as optimistic over the long term.

T-cell lymphoma is often cutaneous, and a preliminarily diagnosis can often be made by visual examination and palpation. The tests that can determine if a cancer is T-cell lymphoma include flow cytometry or immunocytochemistry (ICC).

CTCL may appear as a chronic rash or a flaky skin allergy with crusts or tumors on or under the skin. Because about 10 percent of CTCLs become systemic over time, treatment should be provided if possible.

The most common CTCL is mycosis fungoides, a low-grade cancer that can be treated topically with ultraviolet light, steroid creams, or topical chemotherapy. Solitary cutaneous lymphoma tumors are surgically removed. If the biopsy finds that cancer cells exist at the perimeter of the biopsy sample and the margins are therefore not clean, a second surgery or follow-up radiation and/or chemotherapy may be recommended. If the margins are narrow but clean, and microscopic disease may or may not remain, then follow-up treatment may or may not be needed.

When there are multiple CTCL tumors in different locations, these may be treated with chemotherapy. Protocols often used include the CCNU (lomustine), CHOP, or COAP protocol. COAP uses the drugs cytoxan, vincristine, cytosine and arabinosine, usually for eight to thirteen months.

According to Dr. Villalobos, providing T-Cyte (a signaling protein that stimulates healthy T-cells) and Hollywood Safflower Oil (3 ml per kg on three consecutive days) has been helpful in some CTCL cases for which she has provided treatment.

Transmissible Venereal Tumors (TVT)

TVT is a tumor that originates in the genital tract of male or female dogs. If the tumor is not visible—for example, it may be hidden inside the vagina or uterus—it may spread and first be noticed on a dog's nose, mouth, anus, or elsewhere. TVTs are generally benign and often regress on their own, but in some cases they progress into malignancy. In an immunosuppressed dog, TVT can spread to the lymph nodes.

TVT is highly contagious via mating, sniffing, licking, or any contact between dogs. Immunosuppressed dogs are at high risk for developing a TVT tumor, if in close contact with a dog that has one.

TVT is very treatable, with a high cure rate and a good prognosis. The treatment is usually chemotherapy with vincristine or doxorubicin. After treatment, tumors can recur.

▷ *Homi Lawrence's Story*
Magic Bullet Fund dog Homi came into the fund in January 2009 with TVT. My friend, Dr. Alice Villalobos, provided chemotherapy for Homi, and he has been in great shape for five years and counting. Here is Homi's story, told by his owner:

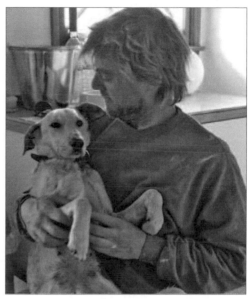

I first saw Homi in February 2008 in Alamos, Mexico, lying in the street sleeping. He was thin but I was told he belonged to a family round the corner. I was busy dealing with other stray-dog-related issues, and wasn't able to do anything to help him.

Imagine my horror when I was back in Alamos in November 2008 and I saw him lying in the road, barely able to get up when cars came by. He had an open wound on his back and looked like a skeleton with dull, lifeless eyes. He had two bloody tumors on his penis. This time I had to do something!

We had to try catch him first, which despite his condition was not easy. Steve finally put some welding gloves on and we managed to use a rope to catch him as he was scared and quite likely to try to bite one of us. My boyfriend and I thought the vet would tell us that Homi had to be euthanized, but to our surprise, he said that he thought Homi had TVT and could be cured completely. Homi started the treatment there and then. After two weeks, the tumor on his back went down significantly. After four weeks, Steve drove back to LA with Homi and our two other rescue dogs.

Two weeks later, blood was dripping from Homi's penis. The tumors were back. It's one thing to have chemo in Mexico, but financially very different in Los Angeles. We took him to Alice Villalobos, DVM, in Woodland Hills, CA, and explained our concerns about the cost of treatment. We thought the only way we could afford more chemo was to take Homi back to Mexico. Dr Villalobos told us about the Magic Bullet Fund and suggested we apply for assistance.

October, 2008: Homi had chemotherapy treatments with assis-

tance from the Magic Bullet Fund. At first we didn't think the treatment was working but the vet decided to try one last blast of a stronger chemo as a final resort. Luckily for Homi (and us), this final treatment worked and finally the cancer was in remission. I can never thank the Magic Bullet Fund enough for what they did for Homi.

April 2014: Homi is extremely well and healthy, thanks to the Magic Bullet Fund. The transformation is unbelievable. The tumors are gone and he has gained weight. His fur has gone from gray and brittle to golden and very soft and shiny. Homi is such a lovely dog—he looks like a different dog!

- Kelly Potter and Steve Lawrence, Hollywood, California

Breast (Mammary) Cancer

Mammary tumors are estimated to occur at a rate of approximately 160 per 100,000 dogs in the population. Every day, roughly 285 dogs are diagnosed with mammary cancer.

Ninety-nine percent of canine mammary cancers are found in females. The risk of cancer for intact (unspayed) females is 26 percent; for those spayed after the first heat cycle, 8 percent; and for those spayed before the first heat, 0.05 percent. In light of these statistics, it is very difficult to justify not spaying a dog.

Of all cancerous tumors in female dogs, half are mammary tumors. Half of these are malignant; the other half are benign. Malignant mammary tumors can be adenocarcinomas, inflammatory carcinomas, sarcomas, or carcinosarcomas. Because benign mammary tumors can grow quite large and are likely to become malignant, all mammary tumors should be surgically removed. Often the glands (breasts) above and below the affected gland are also removed. Local lymph nodes may also be removed if metastasis has occurred.

A mastectomy is performed if tissue outside of the nodule contains cancerous cells. In a radical mastectomy, all glands and the inguinal and axillary lymph nodes are removed. There are five glands on each side of the body. This is major surgery, but less invasive than a human mastectomy. Recovery time is usually about two weeks. If complete excision is not possible, surgery may be followed by chemotherapy.

Generally an unspayed dog is spayed during surgery for mammary cancer. This seems to greatly improve survival times.

The prognosis is good if the tumor is self-contained and is completely excised. Prognosis worsens according to the extent that cancer cells have metastasized (spread) or invaded blood or lymphatic vessels.

Bone Cancers

The most common bone cancers in dogs are osteosarcoma, chondrosarcoma, and fibrosarcoma. About 80 percent are osteosarcoma. An estimated six out of 100,000 dogs develop osteosarcoma, with about twenty-two dogs diagnosed every day in the United States.

Osteosarcoma (OSA)

OSA most often appears in the leg and most commonly develops in large or giant breed dogs, but can occur in any bone of any size dog. Deciding on a treatment plan for this cancer is exceptionally difficult. Osteosarcoma is notoriously predictable for metastasizing quickly to the lungs. Once metastasis to the lungs has occurred, the expected survival is a few months to a year.

A better prognosis is shown in an article published by *PLOS*, August, 2012, titled "Genomic Instability and Telomere Fusion of Canine Osteosarcoma Cells." According to this study, 72 percent of dogs with OSA die as a result of metastasis within two years of diagnosis.

When osteosarcoma is in a leg, the standard primary treatment is amputation. Leg-sparing surgery can be performed instead, for dogs who cannot tolerate amputation due to obesity, hip dysplasia, weakness in another leg, advanced age or other health issues. Leg-sparing surgery is also chosen rather than amputation for owners who are emotionally unable to have their dog's leg amputated.

If metastasis is suspected, leg-sparing surgery is palliative. If there is a chance that metastasis has *not* begun, and the owner wants to give the dog a chance to be in the small percentage of dogs with osteosarcoma who survive more than one or two years, amputation allows for this possibility.

Before amputation, a three-view radiograph (x-ray) is taken of the lungs. This is done no more than a day or two before surgery. Don't agree to x-rays before you decide on a surgery date. If there is a time lapse between x-ray and surgery, the x-ray will have to be repeated.

In 2009, I had a conversation with Dr. John Farrelly DVM, ACVIM (Oncology), ACVR (Radiation Oncology). He was then Head of Radiation Therapy at The Animal Medical Center in New York City. Dr. Farrelly He said that for dogs with OSA in a limb, in 90 percent of cases, by the time diagnosis and amputation occur, the cancer has already begun to metastasize to the lungs.

In many cases, metastasis is not found in the lungs on the pre-surgery x-ray, even though metastasis has begun. It is not found because at early stages, tumors in the lungs are so small that they are undetectable by any testing methods. These miniscule tumors are called "micro-mets" (microscopic metastases). They may be detectable only by bone scan.

When studies show that the cancer has metastasized to the lungs, amputation surgery is canceled. Amputation is not done if the cancer has spread to the lungs because the dog may spend his last few months recovering from surgery and adapting to life on three legs. When amputation is not an option, palliative radiation treatments may reduce the size of the tumor and reduce bone pain. Chemotherapy has little or no benefit.

Amputation may be followed by chemotherapy in an effort to hinder metastasis to the lungs that may be in progress. The standard course of chemotherapy for dogs with osteosarcoma is alternating treatments with the drugs doxorubicin and carboplatin. However, cancer metastasizing to the lungs cannot be stopped. There are studies underway for treatments that stop or slow the progress, but to date there are no treatments available. Many owners opt for amputation and then allow their dogs to have a high quality of life without follow up treatments that promise very little or no additional survival time.

Your veterinarian may want to see your dog for periodic x-rays, to find out if the cancer is spreading to the lungs. If it is, there is nothing that can be done to stop it, so checking periodically has no value. You will eventually (within months) see your dog panting, become unable to take long walks, and have difficulty breathing.

An owner can choose to give the chemotherapy treatments (several alternating treatments with doxorubicin and carboplatin, or six treatments of carboplatin), or not to give the follow-up treatments. An owner can choose to take their dog to the clinic for periodic x-ray or Ultra Sound studies or not to.

Those hoping to cure osteosarcoma in their dog must amputate as early as possible and pray that the cancer cells have not yet begun to migrate to the lungs. Average survival time is six months to a year, whether follow-up chemotherapy is given or not. Amputation is done with cautious optimism, in a very hopeful attempt to beat the odds.

In those lucky few, when amputation occurs before the cancer has begun to metastasize, the dog can have a normal, healthy life on three legs. Yes, normal! To the amazement of owners, most dogs recover from surgery and resume their normal activities very quickly. In fact, the procedure is usually much more difficult for the owner than it is for the dog.

▷ **Bullit Clark's Story**

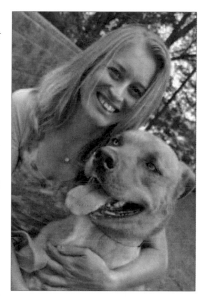

Bullit found me when he was just five weeks old. I named him Bullit after Steve McQueen's movie. In Boulder, Colorado, we hiked mountain peaks, took naps in shady parks, and sat by rivers and streams.

Our world changed in December 2009 as I returned home from a visit with family. Bullit was limping on his left front leg. The vet took x-rays to rule out osteosarcoma.

Veterinary oncologist Dr. Ehrhart sat with me and gave me the news confirming Bullit's cancer diagnosis. She spent a lot of time with me going over every treatment option in detail: Amputation only, amputation plus chemo, radiation.

She told me that whatever decision I made for Bullit was the right decision, that there was no wrong decision.

I decided I wanted as much time as possible with Bullit and that meant amputation. But how was I going to afford this surgery? I applied to Magic Bullet Fund for assistance. When Laurie Kaplan *called to say that the fund would help us I sobbed tears of joy.*

We scheduled Bullit's surgery four days later. Bullit recovered from the surgery like a champion. I nursed his incision carefully and followed instructions precisely. He rebounded on three legs incredibly. I think it was harder on me than it was on Bullit.

After the amputation Bullit had four chemotherapy treatments. While the oncologist had assured me that whatever treatment path I chose would be the right one, the vets highly recommended giving Bullit chemo after the surgery because microscopic disease may remain.

Bullit and I continued with our hiking and camping adventures. I gradually increased his walking time and let him tell me when he was tired. He slowed down a little with three legs, but his spirit continued. He still loved being out on the trails with me, taking breaks to soak up the sun.

Bullit lived happily as a tripawd doggie for nearly four and a half years. I am so grateful to the Magic Bullet Fund for giving us more time together. In April 2014, there was a new tumor in his other leg. We spent Bullit's last days enjoying the great outdoors, car rides to the parks and one last road trip to Salida.

Bullit passed away peacefully last Thursday night, June 12, 2014. I held him tightly in my arms while he drifted off. I whispered in his ear, and told him how grateful I was that he chose me as his guardian. I felt him take his last breath as he crossed the Rainbow Bridge. Now I walk the earth alone, knowing in my heart that his spirit is watching over me.

–Molly Clark, Boulder, Colorado

If you think that life for a three-legged dog (a tripod) is hard or unhappy, don't tell the dogs that! Tripod dogs generally spend one night in the hospital after amputation and go home the following day.

Within a few days, they learn to balance on three legs, run, jump, and go up and down stairs. Their mobility continues to improve as the muscles build in their three remaining legs. The time it takes a dog to adapt to life on three legs after amputation is dependent on the dog's size (smaller dogs learn to balance more easily), age and health.

A dog recently in the Magic Bullet Fund, Lulu, had a malignant tumor in her leg. Before applying for assistance, Lulu had surgery but the surgeon was not able to remove the entire tumor. Lulu's owner was understandably concerned about the cancer spreading, and was seeking assistance for chemotherapy treatments. Since Lulu was young and healthy other than the tumor, I asked the owner if she had discussed amputation with her veterinarian. She had, but felt that this was not an option for Lulu. I could not imagine why and was surprised by her answer. Lulu is blind.

Chondrosarcoma

The bone cancer called chondrosarcoma is a tumor that develops in the tissues *on* the bone rather than *in* the bone. Chondrosarcoma has a much better prognosis than osteosarcoma. It does not tend to metastasize to the lungs and does not progress as quickly as osteosarcoma. Ten percent of all bone tumors are chondrosarcomas. The incidence of this cancer is less than one per 100,000 dogs.

When chondrosarcoma is on a bone in a leg, the recommendation is often amputation. If metastasis has not begun and the entire tumor is removed, then the cancer is gone, although a new tumor may develop at any time.

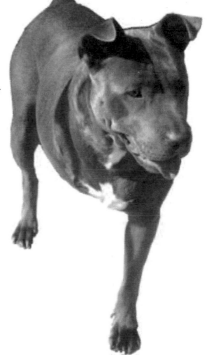

▷ *Lou's Story (anonymous)*

Lou was diagnosed with chondrosarcoma at one and a half years old. I was at work when we got the call from the vet. I absolutely crumbled and burst into tears. It was total shock and devastation.

March 8, 2007, we drove three hours to the surgeon and Lou's right front leg was amputated. He called me later to say that Lou was in recovery and doing well. I did not sleep much that night.

We picked Lou up the next morning, less than twelve hours after the surgery. I was scared, anxious, excited, sad, and nervous all at the same time. To our surprise and amazement, Lou walked out to us in the waiting room! We laughed and cried. She walked to the car too, but I had to lift her in.

We do not know what we would have done without Laurie and the Magic Bullet Fund. They gave us financial support, and so much information. I do not think I would've stayed sane without Laurie's support.

Update from Lou's Aunt: *Lou had a wonderful quality of life until the middle of 2013. At eight years old, she declined rapidly and we suspect that the cancer had returned. Lou was put to sleep on December 31, 2013.*

In the Magic Bullet Fund, we always strive to give the dogs at least one additional year. Many of the dogs we help are seniors so we don't often get to give a dog more than a year or two. Occasionally, we have the opportunity to give a young dog like Lou the amazing gift of surviving many additional years.

Lou recovered very well, and adjusted immediately to having only three legs. She could run just as fast as she did with four legs! Lou's owner called on the phone frequently and had Lou sing "I love you" to me.

Cancers of the Blood

Often, cancers that end with "oma" are benign and those that end with "sarcoma" are malignant. Because dogs do not get the non-malignant (benign) form of lymphoma called Hodgkin's disease, the terms "lymphoma" and "lymphosarcoma" are synonymous.

Multicentric Lymphoma; Lymphosarcoma (LSA)

Multicentric lymphoma is primarily in the lymph nodes. With other cancers, when the cancer spreads to the lymph nodes it is considered to have metastasized. But in multicentric lymphoma, when the cancer has spread outside of the nodes (extra-nodal) or to the liver or spleen, then it has metastasized. At stage V, the cancer is affecting the bone marrow and is very difficult to treat successfully.

Types of lymphoma other than multicentric and cutaneous include mediastinal lymphoma in the chest cavity (which causes coughing and eventually inhibits the dog's ability to breathe), alimentary or gastrointestinal lymphoma (which causes vomiting, diarrhea, and weight loss), ocular lymphoma, and central nervous system lymphoma.

Philip Bergman, DVM, MS, PhD, ACVIM and Chief Medical Officer for BrightHeart Veterinary Centers, says, "Lymphoma is the third most common cancer found in dogs, with an incidence of twenty-four cases per 100,000 dogs per year." Every day, more than 1,500 dogs are diagnosed with lymphoma. An article in *Veterinary Oncology Secrets* (editor Robert C. Rosenthal, DVM, PhD) estimates the annual incidence of canine lymphoma at 110 cases per 100,000 dogs. This would mean that each day, more than 7,000 dogs are diagnosed with lymphoma.

Keep in mind that these statistics include only reported cases. Cancer is not a reportable disease in dogs, as it is in humans. Of pets with cancer, those that receive treatment may be reported in one manner or another. Those that are not treated with surgery, chemotherapy or radiation therapy are generally not reported at all.

Lymphoma is a very aggressive cancer. Most dogs appear to be so strong and healthy when diagnosed, that the owners are shocked and find it hard to believe that their dog has such a deadly disease. Lymphoma progresses very quickly, with an expected survival (without treatment) of only four to eight weeks.

But lymphoma is also highly treatable. Treatment for most canine cancers offers a limited or variable success rate. With chemotherapy, 80 to 90 percent of dogs achieve remission quickly, and those dogs have a very good chance at holding remission for twelve to eighteen months. Veterinary oncologist Susan M Cotter DVM, DACVIM (Small Animal Internal Medicine and Oncology), Distinguished Professor of Clinical Sciences Emerita at Tufts, says, "Dogs with lymphoma have an average survival of around a year past diagnosis, with a good quality of life."

Diagnosis through fine-needle aspirate (FNA) is a good first step but should be confirmed with a surgical biopsy, in which a small slice of a lymph node is removed and analyzed.

Occasionally, the diagnosis is still unclear after FNA and surgical biopsy. Treatment can begin without a definitive diagnosis, or polymerase chain reach (PCR) may be used to obtain a firm diagnosis. In PCR, a sample of DNA is duplicated many times over, to maximize and make more visible the lymphocytic material in the sample.

There are many tests that can be done, such as typing, subtyping, staging, and grading. In most cases, a veterinarian who has experience diagnosing and treating canine cancer can make a highly educated guess as to which type of lymphoma is present. There are often signs when lymphoma is not B-cell multicentric lymphoma. There may be tumors on the skin, an absence of enlarged lymph nodes, or the dog does not respond to traditional treatment.

If there is no reason to believe it's not B-cell multicentric lymphoma, many veterinarians proceed on the assumption that it is. The alternative is to pursue confirmation via time-consuming and expensive tests (which aren't any fun for the dog, either!).

If there is no evidence that the cancer has invaded any organs, the B-cell lymphoma is most likely stage I to stage IV. Dr. Ruslander Veterinary oncologist at the Veterinary Specialty Hospital of the Carolinas, in Cary, NC, said that in canine lymphoma, "The stage of the disease does not necessarily determine the potential success of treatment unless there's stage V extranodal or bone marrow involvement" (phone call, 2003). Treatment has a good chance of being successful as long as the cancer has not spread to organs, and as long as the bone marrow has not been affected.

A veterinarian may suggest beginning steroid therapy, such as prednisone, when lymphoma is suspected. Steroid therapy is given as part of most chemotherapy protocols. It is also offered as palliative care when chemotherapy is not going to be administered, to slow down the progression of the cancer and afford the dog some extra time. When a dog has been given steroid therapy (such as prednisone) without chemotherapy for two weeks or more, multidrug resistance can prevent chemotherapy from being effective. See Multidrug Resistance, page 121.

Dr. Ruslander says that of dogs with lymphoma given chemotherapy, approximately 5 to 10 percent achieve a cure. Knowing that the disease is considered terminal, I asked what constitutes a "cure." Dr. Ruslander responded, "There is a cure when the tumors do not return." In lymphoma, enlarged lymph nodes are described as tumors.

When you hear the prognosis, your dog's expected survival time, or the expected duration of remission, remember that these are only statistics. There are no guarantees as to which dogs will be in the 80 percent that go into remission. And once remission is achieved, there are no guarantees as to which dogs will not tolerate or respond to treatment, and which will survive longer than the twelve to eighteen statistical months. Chemotherapy for dogs with lymphoma is a roll of the dice. For a young or middle-aged dog in good health (other than having lymphoma), many feel that the odds are good enough to make it worth giving their dog a shot at survival.

If your dog has lymphoma and you are going to provide chemotherapy, begin as soon as possible. Until remission is achieved, active cancer cells are busy progressing, and damaging the body's vital organs. Many of the cancer-fighting agents used in chemotherapy can themselves cause damage to these organs and to the heart. Once the damage is done, the dog, owner, and veterinarian are left with not only the cancer to combat, but organ damage or dysfunction as well.

The healthier a dog's organs are at the start of chemotherapy, the better able that dog will be to tolerate the internal maelstrom that chemotherapy creates. With a diagnosis of cancer, we'd all prefer to hear "early stage," but whenever the disease is discovered is when you begin. It isn't possible to go back in time and discover it earlier, so do what you can starting now.

If your dog has lymphoma, check his lymph nodes every day. See the Lymph Node Locator, page 18, and ask your veterinarian to show you how to find your dog's nodes. If a dog's lymph nodes were enlarged when lymphoma was discovered, those same nodes can be used to gauge remission. When those lymph nodes are no longer enlarged and are difficult to feel, and no other lymph nodes are enlarged, a dog is in clinical remission. When they become enlarged again, he is out of remission.

By definition, a remission is only temporary. After chemotherapy and remission, most dogs with lymphoma are expected to relapse after twelve to eighteen months, but the relapse can happen at any time. Some dogs do not go into remission at all, some come out of remission only two or three months after the protocol ends, or only a few weeks after it begins. Many relapse after the average remission duration of twelve to eighteen months, but others stay in remission for four years or more. Simply feeling the size of the nodes is the best way for you to check daily that your dog is still in clinical remission.

There is a test for cellular or molecular remission. It tests for minimal residual disease (MRD), and it provides information that may be helpful to predict, with some degree of certainty, that a relapse is coming shortly before it becomes apparent via enlarged lymph nodes.

Many of the families in the Magic Bullet Fund whose veterinarians have used this test have been disappointed. Some have celebrated when the test confirmed that their dog was in molecular remission, only to see the cancer return soon thereafter and claim their dog's life. Others have begun to grieve for their dog when the test indicated a relapse, and then watched their dog survive, in remission, for quite a long time.

In dogs with multicentric lymphoma, the lymph nodes usually enlarge quickly when remission is lost. Checking the size of the lymph nodes and finding them to be small is probably the best confirmation that a dog is still in remission.

If your dog has been diagnosed with lymphoma and treatment is not effective, it is possible that the underlying disease is actually leukemia. This cancer can be difficult to diagnose and is often initially misdiagnosed as lymphoma, only to be re-diagnosed as leukemia after chemotherapy treatments have been given but the dog does not go into remission. A complete blood count (CBC) and a bone marrow aspirate (with anesthesia) are used to diagnose leukemia.

Leukemia

This cancer arises from cells in the bone marrow. Leukemia is relatively rare in dogs and carries a poorer prognosis than other types of cancer.

When chemotherapy treatments are provided for other cancers, it is known that the drugs may damage the bone marrow and an effort is made to provide enough chemo to kill the cancer but not enough to damage the bone marrow. Since leukemia is a cancer of the blood that originates in the bone marrow, and since a dog cannot survive when the bone marrow is not functioning. fighting cancer of the bone marrow is difficult.

Acute lymphoblastic leukemia can be treated with chemotherapy. The expected survival is six months to two years. Chronic lymphocytic leukemia progresses more slowly and is often not treated until there are symptoms, or until a CBC shows that the bone marrow is not producing new blood cells properly.

▷ **Oliver Colangelo's Story**

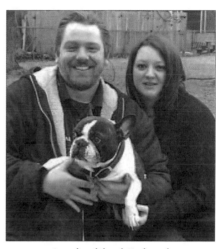

Oliver was a sweet, loving French Bulldog. He was mischievous, playful and a joy to be around. I would wake up in the morning to find him laying on my chest with his face right up to mine, snorting.

At the beach in Michigan's Eastern Upper Peninsula, Ollie ran off leash and swam. French Bulldogs aren't big on swimming, but Ollie was a brave little guy. I'm not saying he liked it, but he braved it for us. The same was true for his cancer.

February 7, 2012 Oliver saw our veterinarian, Dr. Scott Butts of Fowlerville Veterinarian Clinic, for what we thought was a back problem. To our shock and dismay, Dr. Butts diagnosed Chronic Lymphocytic Leukemia and referred us to the Animal Cancer and Imaging Center.

Dr. Jessica Ottnod gave us a treatment plan and an estimate. Oliver was so sick, and without treatment we would have only had a few weeks left with him, but I had recently been out-sourced from my job with Ford Motor Company and we had very little resources. So, the clinic provided information about the Magic Bullet Fund. We were so blessed and are grateful to this day for the Fund's help and support.

In February 2012, Oliver was treated with prednisone, Adriamycin, Vincristine and Cytoxan, and then CCNU. Nothing was working. Then he was switched to a human chemo drug called Hydroxyurea. This turned out to be a great medication for Oliver and he did very well on it. We needed to take care while handling the drug, wearing gloves and watching where he urinated, but it was worth it. Oliver had very few symptoms. He did lose some hair in patches, but other than that you would have never guessed he had cancer. He was a tough little guy.

We had Oliver for almost a year past his diagnosis and lost him November 22, 2012, on Thanksgiving Day. He had developed swelling in his lymph nodes that obstructed his airway along with fluid in his lungs and was unable to rest because of difficulty breathing.

When life became too much for our little buddy to bear, we took him to an emergency vet where he was given oxygen to make him comfortable. We stayed with him for a while, and we were by his side when he crossed to the Rainbow Bridge.

The following weeks were dark in our home. Then, out of the blue, we were presented the option of rescuing another French Bulldog. We knew that if Oliver was out there, and he could, he would give this little dog in need the thing he loved the most in the world—us. We adopted her without hesitation, and she brought joy back to our lives. I believe that was Oliver's wish for us.

- Michelle Colangelo, Livonia, Michigan

Hemangiosarcoma (HSA)

Of all tumors in dogs, only about 6 percent are hemangiosarcomas. This cancer occurs more in dogs than in any other species. This is a very aggressive high-grade soft tissue sarcoma. It originates in cells found in the lining of blood vessels. There is no successful treatment for this cancer.

There are few or no early symptoms that a dog owner might notice and act on. The cancer is often so advanced when discovered that there is no time for treatment to be given. For splenic hemangiosarcoma, surgery to remove the spleen can provide three weeks to six months survival. If this is done early, before any metastasis has occurred, survival is possible.

Surgery may be followed by chemotherapy and immunotherapy. Follow-up chemotherapy may double the survival time, but if metastasis has begun before surgery, chemotherapy may only provide an extra month or two of survival.

If a dog has surgery as soon as the cancer is discovered and survives hemangiosarcoma for more than four to six months (with or without chemotherapy), then most likely the surgery was done early enough to remove the cancer entirely, before metastasis began. Survival longer than the expected four to six months is dependent on luckily discovering the hemangiosarcoma early, and finding that the tumor can be completely surgically removed.

Hemangiosarcoma eventually causes fatal "bleeding out." The Chinese herb Yunan paio (or Yunan paiyo, Yunnan baiyao, Yunnan bai yao (or any combination of these) has been found to be very helpful for dogs with hemangiosarcoma. It has been shown to control the bleeding out to some extent and for some length of time. Many veterinarians recommend Yunan paiyo for their patients with hemangiosarcoma.

The University of Pennsylvania School of Veterinary Medicine compounded a mushroom-based Chinese herbal called I'm-Yunity, thought to help dogs with hemangiosarcoma of the spleen. In 2012 a clinical trial was funded by a grant from Chinese Medicine Holdings LTD and was conducted by Dorothy Cimino Brown, professor and chair of the Department of Clinical Studies and director of the Veterinary Clinical Investigation Center, and Jennifer Reetz, attending radiologist in the Department of Clinical Studies.

The results of this trial are found in an article in *Evidence-Based Complementary and Alternative Medicine* (Volume 2012, Article ID 384301) titled "Single Agent Polysaccharopeptide Delays Metastases and Improves Survival in Naturally Occurring Hemangiosarcoma."

"We were shocked," Cimino Brown said. "Prior to this, the longest reported median survival time of dogs with hemangiosarcoma of the spleen that underwent no further treatment was 86 days. We had dogs that lived beyond a year with nothing other than this mushroom as treatment."

▷ *Tushka Berthold's Story*

In 2005, a gentleman in South Carolina called me, crying so hard I could hardly understand him. His Siberian husky champion, Tushka, had hemangiosarcoma, and he needed help.

He had me overnight the first edition of this book to him. We discussed diet and supplements, and alternative treatments.

I asked him to contact Dr. Villalobos, who helped the man and his wife with more suggestions about treatments and supplements. He consulted several other veterinarians and used every holistic and alter-

49

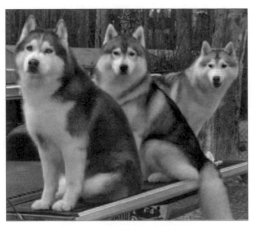

native treatment he could find.

Despite all efforts, this beautiful dog did not live beyond the expected four-month survival time.

A year later, the owner called again. The champion's brother had the same cancer. Again we had consultations and the dog had a series of traditional and alternative treatments, but again we failed to reach a survival of more than a few months.

- Laurie Kaplan

Squirt, Tushka and Spicee

Multiple Cancers

While reviewing applications to the fund, I often notice trends in the diagnoses. In 2010 there was a sudden rash of applications for dogs diagnosed with two types of cancer simultaneously. The most common combination was lymphoma and mast cell cancer.

"Multiple primary cancers" does not include a cancer that has metastasized to other regions or organs. For example, bone cancer will generally metastasize to the lungs. When it does, there is cancer in the leg and in the lungs, but they are not two different cancers. The cancer in the leg is primary bone cancer, and the cancer in the lungs is secondary bone cancer. Metastasized or secondary cancer is often found in the lungs, lymph nodes, or spleen.

If a dog has one type of cancer that is active (not in remission), it's unusual for a second type of cancer to develop. It is as though the cancer stakes a claim, becomes territorial, and destroys developing cells if another type of cancer attempts to move in.

For about two years, in 2010 and 2011, I noted a rash of multiple cancer diagnoses in dogs and just as suddenly, they disappeared. In the past four years there have been none. The only possible explanation I can find is misdiagnosis and over-diagnosis due to an over-zealous concentration on diagnosing and treating cancer in pets.

Multiple simultaneous cancer is unusual but not impossible. When more than one cancer is present, a difficult decision has to be made concerning whether or not to treat both cancers simultaneously. In some cases a chemo protocol can be found that treats both cancers. If surgery is needed for one of the cancers, then chemo is usually halted until two weeks after the surgery. If the treatments cannot be combined, then the condition most likely to become fatal sooner is the one that is treated.

▷ *Miles Gregory's Story*

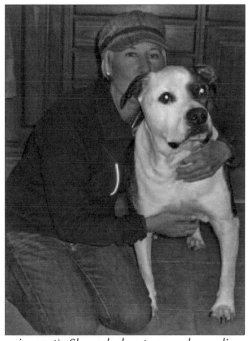

Everyone who met Miles was captivated by his smile and good nature. He was sensitive, sweet, calm, and easy going. We called him Mr. Miles since he was a puppy, since it always fit his style.

Mr. Miles was scheduled for ACL surgery on July 28, 2012. On the day of surgery, however, his white and red blood cell counts were elevated and they couldn't perform the operation. Veterinary oncologist Dr. Erin Bannink performed countless tests (which added up in cost). She ruled out several conditions and then came to the conclusion that Miles had chronic leukemia.

August 15th 2012, Miles' cancer treatment with prednisone and Leukeran began. Miles stayed on the medicine and had monthly checkups from then on. We were extremely blessed that he did well for such a long time. His blood counts were good, his energy level and quality of life were wonderful for a whole year.

We researched what type of food to feed him. We changed his diet to all organic and wished we had done that earlier. We exercised him and made sure he was well rested and not stressed. We found that we could get Leukeran less expensively through a Canadian pharmacy called Rx Canada Direct. Then we got help from the Magic Bullet Fund and we were able to continue his treatment until the end.

In August 2013, a bruise-like formation appeared suddenly on Mr. Miles' belly. Dr. Bannink did more testing and the results were heart wrenching. Mr. Miles had another cancer—lymphoma. We stopped the Leukeran, since it wasn't helping anymore. Mr. Miles was getting swollen lymph nodes all around his neck and head.

There was nothing more to do for Mr. Miles. Fighting two types of cancer was just too much. It was one of the hardest times in my life. I was starting my nursing school program then, trying to study, work, and care for my sweet boy. Miles was family to me, and always will be.

Within a few days, he stopped eating. After three days of fixing all his favorite foods, I knew it was time to stop his suffering. On October 18, 2013 our vet came to our home to peacefully send sweet Mr. Miles home to God and the Rainbow Bridge. One day I know we will be back together. Until then, I think of him daily and always with love.
- Jill Gregory, Fenton, Michigan

3

Your First Decisions

Dog owners are often shocked when their veterinarian says the word "cancer." In many cases, a dog is not acting sick and does not look sick. It is difficult to believe that this strong, healthy animal has a deadly disease. Before you even have a chance to absorb the idea of your dog having cancer, you will be asked to make decisions about diagnostic testing.

A diagnosis is needed before any treatment plan can be formulated. The diagnosis will tell you whether or not your dog has cancer. If there is a mass, it will tell you if the mass is cancer or not, and if it is benign or not. If it is cancer, the diagnosis may also tell you the stage and grade.

A veterinarian may be able to establish a preliminary diagnosis of a mass or tumor based on observation and a hands-on examination. Before treatment can begin, a definitive diagnosis is necessary. It is always important to find out the type of cancer. In some (but not all) cases, it is also important to find out the type, stage, and/or grade of the cancer. With this diagnostic information, a veterinarian can determine which treatment plan will have the best chance of fighting that particular cancer.

There are many diagnostic tests that can be done. Some tests will help determine the best way to provide treatment whereas others may be useful for gathering academic information but will not benefit your dog. If you are not planning to provide cancer treatment due to your dog's age, health, or due to financial constraints, there is no need to have any tests at all done.

Your veterinarian will draw blood for a CBC and a Chemistry Panel. If you can feel the mass with your fingers, the veterinarian may attempt FNA (Fine Needle Aspirate), or may remove a bit of tissue from the tumor via Tru-Cut® tissue biopsy. FNA is a very simple and quick procedure generally done without anesthesia. Cells are extracted from the mass through a needle and studied under a microscope, to determine if cancer cells are present.

The information obtained from FNA may not be sufficient for a firm diagnosis, but an attempt at FNA is still worthwhile. FNA is less invasive, less traumatic, and less expensive than a surgical biopsy. It may yield a preliminary diagnosis, or it may rule out cancer, in which case your veterinarian will look for a different cause for your dog's symptoms.

FNA may fail to extract cells, when the tumor is solid and contains no fluid to be extracted through a needle; or when the needle was not inserted into the tumor (missed it). When FNA fails to extract cancer cells, but cancer is suspected, the next step is an incisional or surgical biopsy.

After an incisional biopsy, your clinic sends the tissue sample to a laboratory, and the laboratory sends a biopsy report to your clinic. Ask for a copy of this report for your dog's medical folder. A biopsy report may name a specific type of cancer found in the tissue sample. Often, however, the report offers a "differential." When the exact cancer type is uncertain, the differential states the best (least destructive) and worst (most aggressive) types of cancer it may be.

If none of the above is successful in diagnosing the mass, a surgical biopsy is the next step. Please read about surgical biopsies in the Chapter "Surgery for Canine Cancer."

What Other Tests are Needed?

Feel free to decline diagnostic tests that will not help your dog. You might decline a test that could rule out a subtype of the cancer your dog has, which is rare and which your dog shows no signs of having. You might decline a test to confirm that your dog does indeed have a subtype that 90 percent of dogs with that type of cancer have.

Some tumors can be diagnosed only via ultrasound, radiography (x-ray), or nuclear scintigraphy (bone scan). Brain and spinal cord tumors can be diagnosed via magnetic resonance imaging (MRI).

When a dog's blood test shows a low count for white blood cells, neutrophils, red blood cells, or platelets, a bone marrow biopsy may be recommended. If the bone marrow's ability to produce new blood cells has been compromised, this becomes the primary issue. Even if the cancer vanishes, a dog cannot survive without a functional bone marrow.

To find out if the bone marrow's ability to produce new blood cells has been compromised, cells in the bone marrow are aspirated. This test is like a fine needle aspirate, but the needle is not fine because the bone has to be penetrated. The large needle is inserted and punched into a bone to extract a sample containing marrow cells from the deep center of the bone. This test should not be preformed unless necessary.

> At the time of Bullet's first chemotherapy treatment, the doctor suggested doing a bone marrow biopsy or aspiration, which would tell us if the cancer had invaded the bone marrow. If so, the prognosis would not be optimistic and chemotherapy might not work. But his white blood cell count and hematocrit were normal, so there was no reason to suspect that the bone marrow had been affected. I asked what purpose this test would serve, and Dr. Porzio explained that it would tell us how advanced the cancer was.
>
> I asked, "Would the results alter Bullet's treatment plan?" He said, "No, not at all." In other words, the result of this test would allow the veterinarian to fine-tune the prognosis, and I would be able to make a note in my datebook on the day that Bullet was expected to come out of remission and then die. Because this test can be uncomfortable or painful and because the result was not going to improve our treatment plan at all, and because I had no interest in putting that date in my calendar, I declined the test.

It may or may not be helpful to find out the stage and grade of a cancer. In some cancers, such as mast cell cancer, the stage is an important determinant of the type of treatment that should be given. In many other cancers, treatment will be the same regardless of the stage. Ask your veterinarian how knowing the stage or grade of your dog's cancer will enable you to choose a more effective treatment plan.

"Stage" describes the appearance of a cancer at the time that it was staged. One staging method, developed by the American Joint Committee on Cancer (AJCC), is called the TNM method. TNM examines three aspects of the cancer: T is the tumor size; N indicates whether or not it has spread to the nearest lymph nodes; and M indicates whether or not the cancer has metastasized.

The TNM staging method isn't helpful in all situations. When a dog has multicentric lymphoma, for example, the cancer cells are, by definition, in the lymph nodes, so "N" is not useful information. In that case, the stages from I to V are based on the spread of the cancer from the lymph nodes to the organs.

A cancer's "grade" is determined by how different the cells look from normal cells. Grading tells how aggressive the cancer is. The more abnormal or differentiated the cells are, the more likely the cancer is to grow and spread quickly, and the higher the grade. High-grade cancers are aggressive and may not respond to treatment or may require more aggressive treatment.

If your vet tells you that your dog has cancer in an organ, such as the stomach or liver, ask what type of cancer it is. For example, "liver cancer" only reveals a location, not a diagnosis. Cancer in an organ may be a secondary cancer that has spread to the organ from elsewhere in the body. Although some organs are most likely to be invaded by certain types of cancer, the location itself does not reveal type, prognosis or the best course of treatment.

If your vet is a test-aholic, you could be in for a very expensive fight against canine cancer. Be selective. Discuss expected results and potential benefits of each test. Discuss the expected discomfort, pain level, or trauma to your dog and the costs to you. If the potential benefits do not outweigh the potential suffering and expense, just say, "No, thank you."

Your veterinarian is obligated to tell you all of the options available to you for your dog's diagnostics and treatment, from the most aggressive approach to the least. You have asked for his expertise and he should share with you all of the information he has. He should tell you about all of the tests that could define your dog's cancer, but should never pressure you.

Gather information from the veterinarians on your team, and do research on the Internet from reliable sites such as vet schools or veterinary associations. Discover which tests are necessary, which tests might benefit your dog, and which can be omitted without compromising your dog's treatment plan.

If you decline a test, your veterinarian might be offended. He might pressure you to perform the test or refuse to treat your dog unless you have a slew of tests performed. We can only hope that most veterinarians would not pressure a client to spend money on unnecessary tests or treatments, but in the real world, a veterinary clinic is a business. Businesses strive to be successful. In the modern animal clinic or hospital, management is there to watch the bottom line. They must justify purchases of state-of-the-art equipment in terms of quickly recuperating the capital expenses from fees paid by clients.. After the equipment cost has been recuperated, the fees will bring in a very nice profit.

Veterinary practice management has become a business field unto itself. Certified Veterinary Practice Management (CVPM) programs teach students how to do many things to improve a practice. They will be hired by a clinic to bring in more revenue.

Among other things, CVPM students are highly trained to teach clinic staff and doctors how to sell services. They teach the staff when to actually say what the cost of a service will be, and when not to. They teach the staff how to phrase offers of services in such a way that will get the highest number of clients to say "Yes, I do want this service." The subtext is that the staff is taught to manage the client for the benefit of the clinic.

Many clinics have become part of a larger, nationwide company and are no longer owned by a veterinarian who practices at that clinic. The management company sets prices and policies and is there to keep an eye on the profit. Do you feel as though your vet used to be there primarily to keep your dog healthy, and now he is there primarily to collect a fee from you? You are not alone.

Your Dog's Cancer Team

You are the Captain of the team providing treatment for your dog. You are paying for a service, and you can make the final decisions about the services provided. Your dog, your money, your decision.

Perhaps the most important decision you will make is your choice of veterinarian and clinic staff to will provide treatment for your dog. Choose your team carefully, based on competence, communication, and cost.

Find a competent oncologist or veterinarian who has lots of experience providing the type of treatment your dog needs. Find a veterinarian with whom you can communicate, who allows you to ask questions, who provides you with the information you need, and who respects your right to make decisions.

Unless you can say that money is no object, call a few local clinics to compare prices. Treatment fees vary significantly from clinic to clinic. Higher fees don't always translate to better medical care. Above-average costs may be explained by high overhead, investments in high-tech diagnostic equipment, investment in a high-priced CVPM, or an ambitious business plan.

See the Appendix for a list of the Schools of Veterinary Medicine. You should be able to find a veterinary oncologist at any of them. There are also many specialty clinics that offer cancer treatment. Ask your veterinarian for a referral, or search the Internet for "Veterinary Oncologist" followed by your city or county or zip code.

There are millions of dogs with cancer in the United States and only about 250 veterinary oncologists. Obviously, it's just not possible for every cancer dog to be treated by an oncologist. To balance supply with demand, many veterinarians have become proficient at cancer treatment.

In many cases, it makes sense to have a dog's cancer treatment provided by a vet who is not a board-certified veterinary oncologist. There are some situations in which a veterinary oncologist would not be selected to treat a dog. A board-certified oncologist's fees are generally higher than a general practice veterinarian's fees, for the same treatment or test. If cost is a factor, call a few local clinics that give oncology treatments, and ask what the estimated fees would be.

Familiarity is especially important if your dog is fearful or aggressive. If your dog is at ease at your general practice clinic, and if they offer the treatment he needs, this would be a good reason to have treatment there.

If you live in a rural area and there is no oncologist near you, that's okay. Look for a general practice veterinarian, or a resident in oncology who has not yet passed the board exam. There will almost certainly be a veterinarian nearby who is expert at providing cancer treatment.

Most general practice vets who provide cancer treatment have a consultant relationship with an oncologist. When a treatment plan is going smoothly, a consultant will not be needed. However, if adjustments have to be made to handle side effects or to achieve a remission, then your veterinarian will contact a specialist for guidance. You may at any time ask your veterinarian to consult a veterinary oncologist.

Many oncologists at veterinary schools or in private practice make themselves available for consultations with non-boarded veterinarians treating dogs with cancer. The specialist can advise your veterinarian of the best treatment plan or the best way to handle side effects or what to do if the first choice treatment plan isn't working.

Another alternative is to take advantage of telemedicine technology. Veterinarians can use telemedicine to get input from board-certified oncologists. Digital x-rays and ultrasound images can be generated on-site and transmitted to a specialist for interpretation and consultation. There is a fee for consultations, which your vet would pass along to you. A few such telemedicine services are PetRays, Idexx/VDIC Telemedicine, and Oncura Partners.

> *In November 2002, Bullet developed a heart condition. It was first detected by Dr. Bruce Hoskins, at Croton Animal Hospital in Croton, NY. There is no cardiologist on staff there, but we were still able to do some initial testing before Bruce referred me to a cardiologist.*
>
> *Bruce, Bullet, and I settled down on a blanket on the floor, and hooked Bullet up with the lead wires and electrodes. The ECG was transmitted by telephone to Cardiopet while I was kissing Bullet's beautiful face.*
>
> *A veterinary cardiologist at Cardiopet interpreted the results and faxed a report to the clinic within twenty-four hours, along with a diagnosis, prognosis, and very explicit treatment recommendations.*

The size and scope of your team is entirely up to you. Don't be afraid to add to and redefine your team whenever you need to. You should have complete confidence in each of your practitioners and consultants. All team members should have expert knowledge in the facet of your dog's treatment to which they contribute.

Your General Practice Veterinarian

Your veterinarian knows your dog's personality and medical history better than any other member of your team. If your veterinarian also offers cancer treatment, and you want her to treat your dog, she should have a relationship with an oncologist consultant who steps in to offer direction and advice when needed.

Veterinary Cancer Specialist

This specialist may provide your dog's cancer treatment and then oversee the case with follow-up visits. Alternatively, this specialist may act as a consultant when and if needed, while your general practice veterinarian provides the treatments.

- Surgeon

If your dog requires surgery, a board-certified surgeon should either perform the surgery or serve as consultant to a non-boarded veterinarian, to provide direction regarding surgical procedures, margins, and aftercare.

- Medical Oncologist

Board Certified specialists in chemotherapy are called medical oncologists. They have access to cutting-edge information about new and modified protocols, and how to handle side effects. If your dog needs chemotherapy, this specialist may provide the treatment or may serve as a consultant for any veterinarian providing chemotherapy for your dog.

- Radiation Oncologist

There are few veterinary facilities that have the equipment needed for radiation therapy. The equipment is very costly to clinics, and the treatments are very costly to dog owners. Find a veterinary radiologist online here www.acvr.org/public/search.

Other Specialists

Secondary or unrelated health problems may arise. These may be side effects to cancer or to treatment, or they may be health issues that any dog can develop. All specialists must be fully informed about your dog's cancer status and treatment.

Holistic Veterinarian

To find a holistic veterinarian in your area, visit www.AHVMA.org and click "Find a Holistic Veterinarian." Or call (410) 569-0795.

Holistic veterinary medicine can enhance and supplement traditional treatments. If you forgo traditional treatment entirely, a holistic veterinarian can serve as your dog's primary veterinarian.

If your general practice veterinarian is holistic, enlist an allopathic (traditional) team member so that you can receive input from both camps.

Some holistic veterinarians are "purists" and will refuse to treat your dog if he is undergoing traditional treatment. Likewise, some traditional veterinarians will refuse to treat your dog if you employ holistic methods. If you wish to use a combination of holistic and traditional therapies, you'll need to find open-minded team members.

Support Group

Your veterinarian may put you in touch with one of his other clients who has a dog with cancer, or you may already know someone fitting this description. Join an online support group! A great deal of information and emotional support is exchanged among owners of cancer dogs at online support groups. (See Resources in Appendix.)

Friends and Family

Seek advice from people who value the life of a dog as you do—people who will help you make a decision that's comfortable for you and right for your dog.

Find a Treatment Plan

Let's say you have decided that you will put your dog through cancer treatment. You can let the veterinarians decide about the treatment plan, or you can play a part in deciding which treatment your dog should be given and how aggressive you want the treatment to be.

If your vet doesn't tell you about more than one treatment option, it may be because he doesn't expect clients to be interested. If you do want the medical information, ask for it. If you want to know about your dog's treatment, and you want to participate in making decisions about the treatment plan, make sure your vet is aware of this. Don't passively nod "okay" when he explains the plan. Ask what other treatment plans might be effective. Ask why he chose that treatment plan. Tell your vet that, with his guidance, you will make decisions about your dog's care.

There is almost always more than one plan to treat any cancer. Consider carefully the options presented to you by your veterinarian or oncologist. A second opinion from another veterinarian can be helpful. If you take a dog with cancer to ten different veterinarians, they should agree on the diagnosis, but they will most likely recommend different treatment plans.

Compare the treatment plans and the prognoses carefully. If both veterinarians recommend the same treatment, do they also predict the same possibility of treatment success? Do they predict the same possibility of cure or remission, and the same survival time? If not, it's up to you to do some more research and discover which prognosis is more accurate and which treatment would give the best result.

Many pet owners hesitate to seek out a second opinion because they fear that their veterinarian will be insulted. If your veterinarian resents your desire for a second opinion, find a new veterinarian. If you are not confident that your vet's diagnosis or recommended treatment plan are the best ones for you and your dog, or if you believe that there could be a better approach to fighting your dog's cancer, get a second opinion. Your dog's life may be at stake.

Ask Your Veterinarian
- ▶ Will the results of this test provide information that could change my dog's treatment plan? If yes, how? (You may be able to make the decision without doing the test.)
- ▶ Could this test help my dog in any other way?
- ▶ Will the test be traumatic or painful for my dog? Is anesthesia needed?
- ▶ How much will the test cost?

You can be an active participant in the decision-making process for your dog's treatment without a degree in veterinary medicine. If you have a limited understanding of cancer treatment for dogs but you want the best chance of success, consult other veterinary oncologists and search for studies published in veterinary journals. Join an online support group. The members generally do not have veterinary degrees, but some do know a great deal about canine cancer and are willing to share their knowledge, experience, and support. Then make an informed decision based on all of the recommendations.

If you would like help sorting through the options and making a decision, I am available for guidance. I help many people make tough decisions about the best way to help their dog fight cancer. ***You can schedule a guidance phone call with me online at www.asklaurie.us.

Some people don't have the inclination or the time to learn about canine cancer diagnosis and treatment. This does not mean they don't love their dog. If "medicalese" is Greek to you and you want to keep it that way, you can leave the decisions in your veterinarian's hands. If he is not a board-certified veterinary oncologist, ask him to consult one. Members of this small and elite group of experts are aware of the most up-to-date information about canine cancer care. You can leave it up to your veterinarian and a specialist to design a solid treatment plan for your dog.

When Should Treatment Begin?

Get treatment started as soon as possible, even if you haven't yet made any long-term decisions. You can switch to a different veterinarian or a different treatment plan later. But do make a move on the cancer right away. Send it a message that you intend to put up a fight.

All types of cancer have the potential to progress and destroy healthy tissue, if left untreated. Without treatment, cancers grow increasingly stronger and more widespread and thus become more difficult to treat. As the disease continues to progress, the prognosis continues to worsen.

Starting treatment early is important in fighting any type of cancer, but especially important when the cancer is osteosarcoma, lymphoma or melanoma. Every day that passes gives osteosarcoma an opportunity to metastasize to the lungs. It metastasizes quickly and after it does, nothing will stop it. Without chemotherapy, lymphoma can be fatal within one to two months.

A decision to begin cancer treatment for your dog does not obligate you to continue the treatments for any particular length of time, or to complete the protocol. There is no contract. You can stop treatment at any time. If chemotherapy is the treatment your dog needs, you can have a few treatments given and then stop. You can hope that those few treatments will give you more time than the veterinarians predicted. You may gain a few extra months with your dog, or more. If surgery is recommended with follow-up chemotherapy or radiation, you can decide to have just the surgery without follow-up treatment, and hope that the surgery alone will set the cancer back and give your dog months or years of quality life.

It is difficult to do less than "everything you can do," but many people do stop treatment due to financial constraints or because their dog has side effects. After some treatment has been given, you can stop treatment and hope that the cancer has been hindered or stopped. There's nothing wrong with giving your dog an extra three, or seven months of life. If you cannot make a decision, keep your options open by startling treatment.

If you are not planning to provide surgery, chemotherapy, or radiation, there is no need to invest in diagnostics. Before you agree to have any tests done, find out what the treatment will cost for the type of cancer that might be found. If you are not able or willing to give treatment, then there is no need for a biopsy.

You may decide to provide palliative care until the cancer progresses. Palliative care does not mean there is nothing for you to do. Bolster his immune system and provide supplements and diet that fight cancer. Keep a close eye on him and use the "Quality of Life Scale" in the Appendix to decide when your dog is no longer enjoying life. Until that day, give your dog the best last days, weeks, or months any dog ever had.

Could It Be a Misdiagnosis?

When a tumor is found to be benign, and is later found to be malignant, this does not necessarily mean it was misdiagnosed. A benign tumor can become malignant.

The type of cancer most often misdiagnosed may be leukemia. This is a very difficult type of cancer to diagnose and is often initially diagnosed as lymphoma. When the standard treatment for lymphoma fails to yield a remission, further testing may reveal that the disease is actually leukemia.

Lymphoma and other cancers are often not diagnosed at the first opportunity. A very common early sign of this cancer is swollen lymph nodes, but swollen lymph nodes can also indicate infection or allergic reactions. For a dog that has a history of allergies, a veterinarian may reasonably assume that the swollen nodes indicate an allergy, and provide antihistamines. When the nodes don't recede after a week, the veterinarian may then find that the dog has lymphoma.

> *Apart from enlarged lymph nodes, Bullet showed no signs at all of being ill when he was diagnosed. This is often the case when dogs are diagnosed, especially with lymphoma. During his chemotherapy protocol, Bullet became ill many times. I knew it was the treatment (not the cancer) that was making him sick.*
>
> *During one of Bullet's episodes with side effects, I found myself thinking, "What if Bullet was misdiagnosed? Am I putting him through treatment—perhaps killing him with it—when he doesn't even have cancer?" This possibility haunted me.*
>
> *I asked Dr. Porzio and Dr. Hoskins about the possibility of a misdiagnosis. They both assured me that there was no chance of this. They reminded me that the surgical biopsy had been evaluated by two different pathologists and that the diagnosis was most definitely accurate.*
>
> *Their certainty saddened me, because it pulled me out of my hopes that he didn't have cancer. But it also forced me to once again face the fact that Bullet really did have lymphoma. It was a disappointment, but it reinforced my resolve to keep fighting without worrying that I was making Bullet suffer for no reason.*

When treatment is not working, people often ask me if it's possible that their dog was misdiagnosed and is being given the wrong treatment. It is possible, particularly if the diagnosis was made after a fine-needle biopsy without a surgical biopsy, but it is not likely. After a surgical biopsy, the odds of a misdiagnosis are slim to none.

Owners put a great deal of love and energy into the battle to try to save their dog's life. They do everything they are supposed to do to help their dog survive. After this investment, it is very hard to accept that treatment isn't working and that the cancer is winning the battle.

4

Your Dog Has Cancer... Now What?

S uddenly your pal, your playful companion, hiking buddy, confi-
dante, and protector (or protectee), has become a cancer patient. You
no longer look at him the same way. Your eyes, your tone of voice,
your posture, and your energy all speak of sadness, pity, fear, and anger
and so many other emotions that are running through you.

Dogs are always sensitive to the energy (vibes) that their humans
project. Don't let your long face be a "downer" for your dog when he's ill,
and especially not when he's feeling well and happy. When an owner is
upset, a dog wonders what he's done wrong. My message is not to *put on* a
happy face, but to actually *have* a happy face and a happy heart. Hold him
close and let his fur absorb your tears on occasion. But, for the main, stay
upbeat and positive and be grateful and full of joy for the time that he has
been with you and because he is with you now. From this moment on,
thoroughly relish every day that you have together and keep reminding
yourself that your best friend is now on borrowed time. Each day is a
precious gift.

You might say, *"How can I pretend to be happy when I'm so sad?"* Don't
pretend! Tend to your dog, do whatever you can to prolong his life and
preserve his quality of life. Use your imagination—even the smallest
contributions that you make to keep him comfortable and happy are
important. When you've done everything you can and there's nothing
more to do, simply sit by his side, pet him, and sing him a song! Bullet
taught me that dogs like being sung to even if the singer can't carry a tune.
If singing is out of the question, then talk to your dog or read him a poem.
The sound of your voice will be soothing to him.

A prognosis is only an educated guess at how long a patient will
survive. Dogs (and people) outlive their prognoses all the time. Sadly,
many do not survive as long as the prognosis predicts. Prognoses about
how long a dog will survive without treatment, as opposed to with treat-

ment, are based on median survival times. The study that yields these statistics may include twenty-five dogs or 500 dogs. The larger the test group, the more weight the prognosis carries. Many statistics given about canine cancer treatments are unofficial, unscientific, based on anecdotal reports comparing only a small group of dogs.

Here's a prognosis: Without chemotherapy, dogs with lymphoma generally perish within one to two months. The accuracy of this prognosis must vary according to how long the dog had lymphoma before it was diagnosed. It will also vary according to how aggressive the dog's lymphoma is.

According to Bullet's oncology consultant, Dr. Ruslander, about 50 percent of dogs with lymphoma that treat with chemotherapy will survive one year or more, and about 25 percent will survive two years or more. The remaining 25 percent will not survive a year.

I was afraid to hope that Bullet might be lucky enough to fall into the minority of dogs that have a long survival. But I sure liked the sound of a one-year remission. Bullet was just past his ninth birthday when diagnosed. A one-year reprieve from lymphoma would afford him a normal life span for a Siberian husky. It would give me a whole year with Bullet.

At Bullet's first chemotherapy treatment, our veterinarian said that he thought Bullet would be very happy when the weather turned cold. I asked (dubiously) if he really thought Bullet would still be here by the next snowfall.

He was still here. Not only for the entire winter, but for the next four winters! Many dogs survive various types of cancer for long periods of time. Some enjoy a normal life span and live on, to die years later from an unrelated cause or from "old age."

A small percentage of dogs outlive their prognoses by a mile. The prognosis for dogs with lymphoma who are given chemotherapy is twelve to eighteen months. But Bullet and many other dogs survived four or five years. Unfortunately, in order to arrive at an average survival of twelve months, there also must be a small percentage of dogs who survive a much shorter length of time.

When you read about your dog's cancer or hear a prognosis from your veterinarian, be optimistic that your dog will fall into the average survival time. Be cautiously optimistic that your dog might be in the small percentage at the top of the curve, and be hopeful that your dog will not be in the percentage for whom treatment fails. Have hope, but make sure that your hopes, optimism, and expectations are realistic.

Treatment Options

After a diagnosis, your veterinarian will recommend diagnostic tests and eventually tell you about treatment options. He will probably recommend one, but he may (and should) explain several. He should allow you to choose. There are factors he is not aware of, such as your intimate knowledge of your dog's personality and tolerance, your family's preferences and your personal finances.

Surgery, chemotherapy, and radiation therapy are the medical interventions most commonly used to fight cancer in dogs (and people). Within each of these treatment modalities, there is more than one approach. Options may include a costly plan and a less expensive plan, or an aggressive plan and a gentler plan. Don't forget that "no treatment" is always an option. Don't be pressured to put your dog through treatment if this is not what you want.

The options may also include new treatments that may prove to be effective, or may not. Take the time to research new treatments. Ask your vet for a printed study. Find out how many dogs were given the treatment, how long they survived and how many had severe side effects.

Clinics that have access to new treatments before other clinics send out press releases and promotional materials to bring in new clients who are looking for the newest, latest and greatest treatments for their dogs with cancer. In some cases, the clinic that offers the well-established most successful treatment may serve you and your dog better.

Don't forget to listen to your dog! If you watch and listen closely, you will sense what he wants and what he needs. You may think he's only capable of communicating that he wants to eat or pee, but if you're listening, he can tell you much more than that. Watch his facial expressions and body language. As your dog's first advocate, make the best decision you can, and don't look back.

Should Your Dog Have Treatment?

Your first decision is whether or not to go ahead with treatment. This can be a very difficult decision to make.

Ask Your Veterinarian

▶ How much time might we gain for my dog? What's the best possible outcome (i.e., cure or length of remission) of this treatment?

▶ What percentage of dogs with this cancer, given this treatment, survive a year? Two years? What studies show these statistics?

▶ How invasive/traumatic would this treatment be for my dog? To what degree would the treatment compromise his quality of life?

▶ What's the worst possible outcome? Is it that the treatment simply won't work, or might my dog have adverse reactions? If so, what are they, and what percentages of dogs have these reactions?

▶ If the treatment isn't successful, what is plan B? (Ask the questions above again, about plan B.)

▶ What is the total cost of this treatment, including all tests and treatments and follow-up visits, if it works? If it doesn't work?

▶ What other treatment options are there to fight this cancer?

Now you have an understanding of what the treatment would be, what it would cost, what the prognosis is, and how treatment would affect your dog. If you have not yet decided whether or not your dog should have treatment, consider all of the following:

Age

If your dog is geriatric, think about how much longer he would be likely to live if he did not have cancer. If he does have treatment, and if treatment is successful, how much longer might he live after treatment?

Health

A dog with preexisting medical issues may not tolerate treatment as well as a healthy dog. If your dog has preexisting conditions, see if there is a gentler, less traumatic treatment option.

Quality of Life

Weigh the chances of treatment success against the possibility and degree of trauma your dog may endure.

Your Gut Instincts

If you have a strong suspicion that medical intervention will not be successful, you may choose to forgo treatment.

Your Personality

Take your psychological makeup into account. Are you prepared to roll up your sleeves, clean up vomit and diarrhea, and possibly watch your dog become too ill to eat for a couple of days?

Financial Considerations

You adopted a pet and made the pledge that we all make: *"I will take care of you for the rest of your life."* But you weren't anticipating that tens of thousands of dollars would be needed for a fight against cancer.

It is difficult to think about finances when making this decision. Are you putting a price on your dog's life? How much time will $1,000 buy him? How much money is it worth to keep him alive three more months, or two years?

Apprehensions

Fighting canine cancer is a roll of the dice. Cancer is unpredictable. We never know in advance if the treatment we choose will work. We will never know if a treatment that we did not choose would have worked.

There are lots of estimates, prognoses, and statistics. Even when there is a good prognosis, there is a chance that the dog will not survive. For some of the dogs in treatment with a poor prognosis, there is a chance of survival.

If you put your dog through cancer treatment and the treatment is not successful, will you regret having spent the money? Will you feel as though you made the wrong choice?

If you decide against treatment, will you regret it? If you don't treat, or you stop treatment and the cancer returns, don't torture yourself by asking "What if ..."

If you decide to decline treatment, you can simply enjoy the time you have left with your dog and let nature take its course. A decision to decline medical treatment does not mean that there's nothing you can do! You can still help your dog fight cancer and be as healthy and happy as possible, for as long as possible. Use information about diet and supplements for a dog with cancer in this book. Try to buy some time, slow down the disease process, and postpone the decline.

There are many factors to weigh
and there is no right answer
except the one that comes from your heart.

Make a decision that won't result in a haunting voice saying "I should have" or "I shouldn't have." Make the best decision you can, and then accept, regardless of the outcome, that it was the best decision. Once you choose a course of action, do not second-guess yourself.

Don't Believe Everything You Read

I hear from many people that when they learned that their dog had cancer, the first thing they did was start to gather information from the Internet. If you research on the net, you will find a ton of information about canine cancer. You will find well-qualified, up-to-date information and current theories about canine cancer treatments, diet, supplements, clinical trials, and holistic treatments.

You will also find lots of information provided by individuals who are well meaning but are not well informed.

Always check the source of the information. Anyone can post anything on the Internet! Information may be clear or misleading, objective or subjective, true or false. Beware of websites that end in ".org" but are not nonprofit and do not offer tax deductions for donations.

To be safe, do your research at websites maintained by schools of veterinary medicine, specialty animal clinics, veterinary cancer organizations, or human cancer organizations such as NIH (National Institutes of Health) and NCI (National Cancer Institute).

Where to Find Good Information on the Internet
▸ Look for articles in veterinary journals.
▸ Look for websites that aren't selling you a product.
▸ Look for websites that are not published by an individual whose dog has or had cancer. Personal stories about someone's dog may contain information based on their own personal experience that sounds similar to your situation but is actually not.

Don't Believe Everything You Hear

Once you tell people that you have a dog with cancer, you will hear many stories. In fact, I predict that any time you tell a person your dog has cancer, they will tell you a story about their dog or a friend's dog with cancer. They may also have advice or warnings for you. Have an open ear because other people's stories will contain bits of information that will help you help your dog fight cancer. But create an imaginary filter in that open ear, because you will also hear bits of information that will not apply to your or your dog's situation, or will simply be inaccurate.

Your veterinarian will tell you his recommendation for how to proceed with diagnostic tests and treatment. If you take your dog to ten different veterinarians, you may very well hear a different recommendation from each veterinarian. They can't all be right! Pressure your doctor to tell you about the other treatment plans available to you. "What else could we do?"

Your clinic might lean toward a treatment plan simply because it is the one they most frequently use. They may recommend a new protocol that has been successful with a handful of dogs, but may later turn out not to be successful for other dogs. They may intend to use a treatment plan that is actually a variation of an existing protocol, for which they or a group of clinics are trying to discover if the results will differ from those obtained using the gold standard treatment plan. If you want your dog to have the gold standard treatment without experimental variations, tell the veterinarian.

Decide if you want the most aggressive treatment (which may or may not be more successful at fighting your dog's cancer, but will be more likely to cause side effects) or a less aggressive plan (which may or may not be just as successful in fighting the cancer but less likely to cause side effects).

Make a list of treatment options, with a column for each. Below each heading, make a list of the pros and cons according to your qualifiers: success rate according to studies in veterinary journals; number of treatments; dosages (at the high or low end of the recommended dosages); toxicity and likelihood of side effects; and cost.

Two years after Bullet's diagnosis I was walking him, happily noting that he was back to his normal, strong, healthy self. A woman stopped to admire him and, as always, Bullet was happy to receive admiration and be petted. The woman told me a story about her beloved dog. She was in tears.

Her vet had told her that her dog had lymphoma. The vet advised her to "put him down," even though he wasn't even sick yet at all. And she did. Veterinarians are not immune from allowing their personal opinions to be a factor when they make treatment recommendations.

I usually told people about Bullet's cancer, but in this case, I didn't. I didn't have the heart to tell her that Bullet had the same cancer that her dog had, and that he had survived it.

Don't Ever Believe "It's Just a Dog"

What is a dog's life worth? The typical pet dog will not grow up, develop a career, and contribute to society. He will not support you in your senior years or take care of you when you become feeble. He won't even bring you a cup of tea when you've got the flu! (My apologies to search-and-rescue dogs, guide dogs, seizure-alert dogs, and all other working dogs for this generalization.)

But dogs will do something very special and rare. They will give unconditional love, loyalty, and companionship. Indeed, a dog will devote his entire existence to the solitary purpose of pleasing the special person or persons in his life. This is the gift of the dog. In return, we must, at the very least, give our dogs love, excellent care, and respect.

Friends and family may disapprove of your efforts to save or prolong your dog's life. Many simply cannot, and will never, understand. They say, *"But it's just a dog!"* Don't let these naysayers sway you, but don't think for a moment that you will sway them. At the very most, you'll only convince them that you're entitled to your (nutty) beliefs about the value of a dog's life. Instead, join a support group to find others who feel as you do.

A popular dog book author states that dogs should not be treated like human family members, and they should not be given treatment for cancer. Should we then not mend their broken legs? Where should we draw the line? Perhaps I will call the author next time my dog is sick, to find out whether or not I should provide treatment.

To me, and surely to most reading this book, our pets are family members, and their lives do have great intrinsic value. We will go to great lengths to preserve that precious life and that beautiful bond.

Are you committed to taking the journey through cancer treatment with your dog? You may decide to shore up your resources and marshal your forces to wage war against your dog's cancer, or to provide palliative care to optimize quality of life and perhaps extend life, or to release him through early euthanasia to spare him any suffering. Whatever you decide, make peace with your decision. You will not err if you make this decision with love and respect for your dog as a valuable, sentient, living creature who is a member of your family, who has given you his all and who has asked so very little in return.

As cancer-dog owners, we are forced to make very difficult decisions about things like surgery, radiation therapy, chemotherapy, palliative care, and euthanasia. None of the options are appealing, but we must choose nonetheless. So long as you decide from your heart and make choices with love and respect, you will make the right decisions.

Keep a Journal

Sharpen your pencil if you like to write! If you don't, do your best to at least keep a simple list of notable events. Use a notebook in which you can write your notations and insert a copy of each test result, blood test, and report. Always ask your clinic for a printout of each report.

Information in your journal may very well save your dog from having to endure side effects unnecessarily. A few months into treatment, you may find yourself trying to remember. Which agent was it that caused that terrible reaction? How long was it before my dog was feeling better the last time this happened? What were his symptoms, and which remedy was it that finally alleviated those symptoms?

What to Include in Your Journal
- ▶ Original report with the diagnosis of cancer
- ▶ Itemized treatment estimate for your dog's treatment plan
- ▶ Medications and supplements and reactions your dog has to them
- ▶ Changes in diet and your dog's response
- ▶ Changes in eating, urination, and defecation habits
- ▶ Changes in your dog's mood or energy level, ability to take long walks or go up and down stairs
- ▶ Names and dates of treatments. Include each chemo treatment with the name of the drug, each radiation treatment, or surgery
- ▶ Side effects and reactions caused by treatment or by cancer
- ▶ All attempts to counteract side effects and reactions; what worked and what didn't
- ▶ Any secondary illnesses and how they were treated

Veterinarians you consult may ask for information such as when you started giving your dog a medication or supplement, at what dose, and how he responded. Your journal may very well help the veterinarian make the most effective recommendations without any delay.

If you decide to provide treatment and fight your dog's cancer, you will launch an attack against the cancer and it will involve a whole team. And you will be the Captain of that team.

A board-certified veterinary oncologist should be included as a member of your team, either as your dog's primary cancer treatment provider, or as a consultant. Decide what role a veterinary oncologist will play on your team based on proximity, cost, and familiarity.

We each have a different method of fortifying ourselves emotionally. Decide to be strong, for your dog's sake and your own. When you feel overwhelmed or emotionally exhausted, make use of your support system. Gather strength from talking to sympathetic family and friends or online support group members about your journey. Take a break from researching. Sit by your dog and do nothing but stroke him for a while.

When it comes to death and dying, I believe that dogs are blessed with ignorance. They don't know that they may die soon or that they have a disease called cancer. Dogs don't regret or complain about what happened yesterday, nor do they anticipate or fear what might happen tomorrow. We humans are not so lucky. We know, we fear, we anticipate, and we project. While caring for your sick dog, resist your natural inclination to dwell on these emotions—to fret over yesterday's decisions or worry about what tomorrow will bring. Be in the moment—emulate your dog!

Every time Bullet went through a bad spell, I wondered if, and hoped that, he was going to recover "this time." I reminded myself, over and over, to remain calm, treat the symptoms, and hope for the best.

> *The journey is an emotionally exhausting roller coaster ride.*
> *Hang on tight and keep saying your new mantra.*
> *Not today, and not without a fight!*

5

Surgery
for Canine Cancer

S urgery is helpful for many different types of cancers, including mast cell tumors, melanoma, mammary cancer, hemangiosarcoma, osteosarcoma, and others. A malignant tumor that is cutaneous (in the skin) or subcutaneous (under the skin) should be removed if possible. Often, the owner's first decision is: *Surgery or no surgery?*

When a tumor is found to be benign, that does not necessarily mean surgery is not needed. Benign tumors can become malignant. For example, lipomas can become liposarcomas. A growing or bleeding mass, whether it is benign or malignant, should always be removed.

You might decline surgery because of your dog's age or health, because of your finances or for another reason. In that case, "no surgery" is your choice and there is no need to have any more diagnostic tests done.

If you feel that your dog cannot tolerate extensive treatment because of his age or health, or if you have limited funds for treatment fees, you can decline treatment or you can limit the treatment. You can decline surgery, or you can approve surgery but decline any further treatment, such as chemotherapy or radiation therapy.

It is difficult to say no, but there are situations in which it is kinder to the dog to decline treatment than to have treatment. We are so completely responsible for every aspect of our dogs' lives that we feel it is our job to save them from every illness.

> *It is our job to keep our dogs healthy and alive.*
> *But sometimes we have to say, "I cannot fix this."*

If you do want to have surgery for your dog, there may be a choice between curative surgery and palliative surgery. *Curative* surgery attempts to eradicate the cancer, whereas *palliative* surgery attempts to improve a dog's quality of life, knowing that the cancer will progress.

Curative Surgery

If curative surgery is possible, its potential success depends on the type, location, stage, and grade of the tumor, and the number of tumors. And, of course, on the skill of the surgeon.

If your vet says that curative surgery is an option for you to consider, do not consider this a guarantee that the surgery will really get rid of the cancer. The surgeon may find during surgery that the tumor is more extensive than expected. The tumor may later recur, or a new tumor may appear even though you signed up for curative surgery.

Sometimes "curative" surgery turns out not to be curative,
even if all known diagnostic testing was done.

The best outcome occurs when the cancer is limited to a single tumor or multiple tumors in a single location. If possible, the tumor should be completely removed with wide margins. *Wide margins* means that all surrounding tissue that may contain stray cancer cells is removed with the tumor. Wide margins are taken in an attempt to achieve *clean margins.*

Removing a tumor with wide margins means removing the entire mass with a two to three centimeter border of visibly healthy tissue around it. This will be a more invasive surgery than removing only the tumor (as in a lumpectomy), but it will increase the chance of success. It will prevent the cancer from metastasizing during the weeks between a first and second surgery, and it will be an attempt to limit the number of surgeries to one.

I have noticed that in human surgery, scar revision surgery is a cosmetic procedure, to improve the appearance of a scar. In veterinary medicine the term has emerged as a second surgery to remove the scar tissue and a swath of adjacent tissue containing cancer cells that were not removed in the first surgery.

When a second surgery is needed, owners ask, *"Why didn't the surgeon take wide margins the first time?"* First, if a mass is suspected to be benign, narrow margins will suffice. The surgeon may not have been trying to take wide margins.

Second, when a mass is close to bone or muscle or a vital organ, it isn't always possible to remove a wide enough swath of tissue to include the entire mass plus wide margins.

Sometimes a surgeon is not able to remove a tumor with wide margins. Narrow margins means that the tumor was removed with a border of clean tissue around the tumor, but there were cancer cells close to the outer edge of the removed tissue. It is possible that stray cancer cells remain in the dog, and further treatment will be needed to prevent the same or new tumors from returning.

Get a second opinion from an oncologist or board-certified surgeon before allowing surgery to be done on a dog with cancer. Let the veterinarian know that you would like him to make every effort to excise the cancer completely, to the best of his ability, in one procedure. Ask him to remove the tumor with wide margins, as though the mass is known to be malignant. If the surgeon is successful, your dog will not need a second surgery, chemotherapy, or radiation.

After surgery, it is likely that you will receive the news that "your dog needs another surgery," or "now we have to give him chemotherapy," or "now he must have radiation therapy." If the goal was to cure the cancer, but the tumor was only partially removed and part of the tumor remains, radiation therapy or chemotherapy or another surgery will be recommended. Additional treatment is more important when the margins are dirty than when they are clean and wide, or clean but narrow.

If an entire tumor is successfully removed, the biopsy report will often state that clean margins were achieved, but "microscopic disease may remain." As discussed above, this also means that microscopic disease may *not* remain. If the cancer has been removed and microscopic disease does not remain, then there is no need for follow-up treatment.

A biopsy of the removed tissue will examine the tumor within the tissue sent to the lab, and will look for the presence of cancer cells from the tumor all the way out to the edges of the tissue. The biopsy report will state how close to the edges (margins) the cancer cells were found.

Palliative Surgery

Palliative surgery is not expected to stop the cancer. It can reduce pain and/or improve a dog's mobility and quality of life, while the cancer runs its course. Palliative surgery is often used to remove a painful tumor or a tumor that is blocking an airway, the intestines, bladder, or any bodily function.

It makes sense to have palliative surgery done only if it does not include a long, painful recovery, and only if it will improve the dog's quality of life for his last weeks or months. When there is a tumor that is causing the dog discomfort or pain, and the tumor is in a location that makes it impossible to remove with wide margins without also removing bone or muscle tissue, it is more difficult for the owner to make a decision.

An owner may choose to have only part of the tumor removed, to make their dog more comfortable and hopefully to slow down the progression of the cancer. This is called "debulking."

Debulking a large tumor is helpful if it will make a dog more comfortable and possibly slow down the progression of the cancer. Debulking can improve the quality of a dog's life and perhaps prolong life, but with no expectations of a cure or a long-term solution.

In some situations, an owner might agree to tumor-removal surgery, who is not planning to provide another surgery, chemotherapy, or radiation therapy. In that case, there is no need for a biopsy.

> I adopted a 10-year-old Black Lab mix called Parker from the local shelter in 2005. When Parker was fourteen, a tumor the size of a caper appeared on his eyelid. Parker was blinking constantly and rubbing his eye with his paw. Clearly, the tumor was bothering him.
>
> Parker's veterinarian, Dr. Bruce Hoskins, examined the tumor and went over the options with me. Without any diagnostic tests (we didn't know what type of cancer, stage, or grade it was), I opted to have it removed with as wide margins as possible, without removing the eye. Dr. Hoskins said that he could safely remove up to one-third of the lid, and we agreed he would remove up to one-third and attempt to remove ethe entire mass. I did not need any diagnostic testing done before the surgery. I did not feel any need to know all there was to know about the mass. I just wanted it taken out.
>
> After a tumor is removed, the tissue is usually sent to a lab for a biopsy. I wanted Parker to have only one surgery and no other treatment for this tumor. Therefore, there was no reason to have a biopsy done after surgery either.
>
> My sweet Parker passed three years later, at seventeen and a half years old. In those three years, the mass never returned.

For many Magic Bullet Fund dogs that had surgery to remove a tumor, the veterinarians stated after surgery that the cancer would most likely return without further treatment. In many of these cases, the owners declined the additional treatment, and the cancer did not return for years, or did not ever return.

During palliative surgery, the veterinarian may be surprised that the entire tumor lifts out and is completely removed. Sometimes a debulking is done and the tumor, although it was only partially removed, does not return for the rest of the dog's life.

Sometimes "palliative" surgery turns out to be curative.

When a surgery is planned to remove a cancerous tumor, it is often preceded by a three-view radiograph (x-ray) of the lungs, because some cancers typically metastasize to the lungs. How quickly metastasis occurs and to what part of the body can be predicted with some degree of confidence according to the type of cancer.

In its very early stages, metastasized (secondary) lung cancer is impossible to diagnose. The tiny tumor, or nodules, appear as "micro-mets" that cannot be discovered at all by any tests.

If metastasis has begun, and tumors are seen in the lungs, then the surgery is usually cancelled. There is no point in making a dog spend the last weeks or months of his life going through recovery from surgery if lung cancer is developing. However, shadows, calcifications, and nodules can all be misdiagnosed as lung tumors, and often are. Consider getting a second reading of the study, to confirm that the cancer is in the lung.

If surgery proceeds despite the presence of lung mets, the surgery is always palliative. Although primary lung cancer can be treated with some success, secondary lung cancer (a cancer that has metastasized to the lungs from someplace else in the body) cannot.

Chemotherapy can be used to fight secondary lung cancer, but metastasized lung cancer usually results in survival of up to a year, whether chemotherapy treatments are given or not. Once cancer has metastasized to the lungs, palliative (hospice, Pawspice, end-of-life) care should begin. The cancer will progress until the dog has so much difficulty breathing that he has no quality of life.

Ask Your Veterinarian

- ▶ Does the vet expect to be able to get clean margins?
- ▶ If margins are clean, what if any additional treatment will your vet recommend after surgery?
- ▶ If the margins are not clean, what treatment will your vet recommend? Another surgery? Chemotherapy? Radiation?
- ▶ Which anesthetics and pain medications will be used during and after surgery?
- ▶ Is an overnight stay necessary? If so, who will be at the clinic overnight? If no one will be there, can you take your dog home overnight? Or should you have the surgery done elsewhere, at a clinic that is staffed overnight? Or can you pay a vet tech to stay overnight?

If your dog needs surgery, ask for a printed, itemized estimate before you schedule the surgery. The estimate should include fees for diagnostic tests that will be needed before surgery, as well as the surgery itself. It may also include follow-up visits to remove sutures and check on the incision, and pain medications that the owner takes home for their dog.

You will probably see a fee for "boarding." Depending on what surgery your dog will have, you may be able to take him home at the end of the day instead of leaving him at the clinic overnight. If you are going to be at home, and if you are comfortable taking care of your dog after surgery, find out if your dog can come home instead of staying in the clinic overnight. Ask if the vet can schedule your dog's surgery early in the day, knowing that you would like to take him home that night if possible.

When an overnight in-hospital stay is recommended, ask if the clinic is attended overnight. When a dog in the Magic Bullet Fund needs an overnight stay after surgery, I ask this question. If necessary, I pay a veterinary technician to spend the night at the clinic and keep an eye on the dog, in case he needs medication or any type of assistance.

Don't be surprised if you see a fee for use of the operating room (hard to understand, since the operating room is part of the clinic). Soon we will be charged for use of the waiting room while we sit and wait for our dogs to be treated. If it's important to conserve money, compare prices at other clinics in your area.

Checklist for Surgery

- ▸ Follow your vet's recommendations regarding your dog's activity, eating and drinking.
- ▸ Watch for signs of infection. If you see any bleeding, redness or swelling at the incision site, notify your vet.
- ▸ Ask your vet if there is anything you can do at home to keep the site clean.
- ▸ Discuss pain control with your vet. If your dog is having surgery that would be painful for a person, you can believe that it will be painful for your dog.
- ▸ What pain medications will you be given to control your dog's pain at home after surgery? Find out what the upper and lower dosages are.

Amputation Surgery

For a tumor in a leg, the treatment plan may be surgery to remove the tumor, or surgery to remove the entire leg. Removing the leg is obviously more aggressive, with a better chance of eradicating the cancer completely.

Amputation surgery is almost always the treatment of choice when the tumor is osteosarcoma (bone cancer) in a limb. Bone cancer metastasizes quickly to the lungs, but a dog may survive in the few (about 10 percent) cases in which surgery removes the tumor entirely before metastasis begins. Amputation is done in hope that the dog will be in the small percentage of dogs that survive this cancer.

If the dog is not in this lucky group of survivors, that doesn't mean that the amputation was done for naught. If a dog is limping or experiencing pain from the tumor in his leg, the amputation will improve his quality of life.

Amputation can spare a dog from experiencing a painful bone fracture. When the tumor is in the bone and the tumor grows, something's gotta give. The bone eventually fractures. At that time, with a dog in excruciating pain, euthanasia is usually necessary.

If your dog has a tumor in his foot or ankle, you may be surprised when your vet recommends amputation of the entire leg. Dogs find it difficult to walk on four legs when one of the legs is much shorter. They fare much better on three legs.

The Tripawds support group at https://www.facebook.com/tripawds provides great information for anyone whose dog may need amputation surgery. Their slogan is "It's better to hop on three legs than to limp on four."

▷ *Jordan Gleeson's Story*

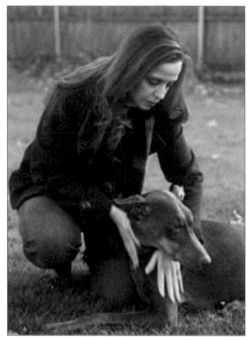

Jordan came into the Magic Bullet Fund with osteosarcoma in August 2010. Amputation surgery was planned, and the surgery went smoothly at Deer Park Animal Hospital in Deer Park, New York.

At 8:00 pm that evening, I received a panicked phone call from Jordan's owner, Karen. The clinic had called her to say that they were closing for the night, and that Jordan would have to be transported—by the owner— to a nearby clinic that was open all night.

I was shocked and furious. Neither of us had been given any advance notice that the semi-conscious Jordan, a few hours after her leg was amputated, would have to be transported. If we had known, of course we would have had the surgery done elsewhere.

I knew Karen would be able to move Jordan, and she did, but at an emotional cost. She is a very strong woman who can do just about anything that needs to be done. But I thought, "What if Karen had gone out of town for the night? What if she was unable for some reason to drive at night?"

Karen and I had many phone calls that night. I called a 24-hour clinic near Karen, New York Veterinary Specialty Center. I made arrangements for Jordan's intake and care, while Karen accomplished the transport. As Karen says, "That was a bad night that formed a forever bond." Karen has since become a volunteer for the Magic Bullet Fund and comes to local events to help me manage the fund's booth.

If your dog is having any type of surgery that requires an over-night stay, please make sure that your clinic is staffed over-night. If it is not, find a clinic that is open and staffed twenty-four hours a day.

- Laurie Kaplan

Checklist for Amputation Surgery

▸ See Checklist for Surgery, above. Be sure to read about metastasis earlier in this chapter.

▸ Often dogs go home the following day, with only a T-shirt. Bandages can tighten due to swelling and cut off circulation. If your dog does need bandages, note how tight the bandages are when you get home. If they become tight, return to the clinic for possible re-bandaging.

▸ Ask your vet to clip all of the hair growing between your dog's toes, and to clip all of his toenails short. This should be done while he is still under anesthesia. He will need all the traction he can get.

▸ Buy a harness with a handle. This is especially important for large dogs. You can use the handle to help your dog up or down stairs, and into or out of the car. You can carry your dog like a suitcase using the handle or just provide a lift so there is less weight on his three legs. Harnesses that are especially good for tripods are the EzyDog® Convert Harness and the Ruffwear® Web Master, both available at www.tripawds.com.

▸ If you have hardwood or ceramic tile floors, buy some rubber-backed mats to arrange for him to walk on.

▸ If your dog will need to go up or down stairs the first few days after surgery, figure out how you will help him, or whom you can call to help.

▸ Join the support group called BoneCancerDogs on Facebook: www.facebook.com/BoneCancerDogsInc.

- ▶ Your dog will find his balance on three legs, and the muscles in those legs will grow stronger. He may not realize that he can't do some things like he used to, so watch him closely at first.
- ▶ Be patient and be vigilant. Limit your dog's activities, even if he wants to run.

For tumors in a leg other than osteosarcoma, amputation may not be necessary, depending on the type of cancer and the location of the tumor.

▷ *Sandy Davis' Story*

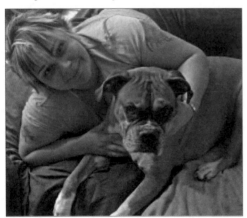

When Sandy was four years old, in 2007, she had a small bump growing on her right arm. We took her to our vet, Dr. Dew, who did an FNA test on the bump. The FNA came back inconclusive and the vet told us to keep an eye on the bump and have it checked again if it grew.

Very slowly, it did grow over the next two years. We brought Sandy back to the vet, who again did an FNA. Again, the test was inconclusive. Again, she said to watch the growth. Another two years went by, and then we noticed it getting quite a bit larger. Now, it seemed to be causing Sandy discomfort.

This time the vet did a surgical biopsy, which came back positive for fibrosarcoma. The vet gave us two options. The first was to remove the tumor with wide margins, followed with chemotherapy if necessary. She did not recommend this option, because she was afraid she would not be able to remove the whole tumor.

The second option was to amputate Sandy's leg. We went to four more veterinarians and they all recommended amputation, to get rid of the cancer completely.

We took Sandy to a veterinary surgery specialist, Dr. Federico Latimer. He also recommended amputation. I finally agreed and prepared myself for this emotionally. I was concerned about how we were going to afford surgery, so I looked for help online. I found the Magic Bullet Fund, I applied, and they said they could help us. I am so grateful to the Magic Bullet Fund for their financial help and emotional support. Sandy would probably not be here today without them.

But when surgery day came, the vet changed his mind. He was concerned that amputation would not be a good idea because of Sandy's weight. We agreed that he would cut out the tumor and a wide margin around it. He said we could try that first and to try to spare Sandy's leg. If the tumor returned we could talk about amputation.

On February 2, 2012, Dr. Latimer removed the tumor completely. There were no traces of cancer left. No chemo treatments were needed; apparently neither was the amputation. Now, in October 2014, Sandy and I are very happy that she still has all four of her legs. In a way, we were very lucky that Sandy is overweight!

- Marisa Davis, West Palm Beach, Florida

Pain Control

Pain control plays an important role in recovery. Cutting through tissue results in pain and can cause tissue-swelling, which can cause pain. Ask your vet if you can apply ice packs to the site. Ice is a wonderful post-surgery tool. In addition to limiting the swelling that occurs, it reduces pain because numbness is always better than pain.

If you are not given pain medication for your dog when you pick him up to take him home, ask for some. Nonsteroidal anti-inflammatory drugs (NSAIDS) may be enough to keep your dog comfortable. But your dog may need more pain relief than NSAIDS provide.

Discuss with your vet which medications should be used, how much to give your dog, and how often. Ask what the upper and lower limits are, in case you find that the dosage is too high (your dog is in a coma) or too low (your dog is crying in pain). A commonly used at home pain medication for dogs is tramadol. This works very well for most dogs, and the dosage can easily be increased or decreased, within the safe range that your veterinarian has explained to you.

Like people, each dog responds differently to medications. For a few days or weeks, depending on how invasive the surgery was, keep a close eye on your dog to evaluate his pain level. Take note of his activities, including eating, drinking, urination and defecation. Your dog should not be crying or unable to sleep at night. At the other extreme, he should not appear to be in a coma. If you feel the medications are too strong or not strong enough, call your clinic and discuss how to adjust the dosage or change to a different medication.

Big Pharma has responded to the explosion in high level caretaking and medical treatment for pets. There are two pharmaceuticals in particular that have been recently marketed for veterinary use and heavily prescribed by veterinarians. In my opinion, these are not appropriately prescribed when used for post-surgery pain.

The Duragesic® pain patch has become very popular among veterinarians for post-surgery pain. This is a transdermal patch that contains a narcotic called fentanyl. The patch has been available for human use for chronic pain patients for many years, but the manufacturer warns specifically, strongly, and repeatedly that it should not be used for short-term pain or for post-surgical pain.

The pharmaceutical insert warns, "Duragesic is contraindicated…In the management of post-operative pain," and "Duragesic should only be used by people who are receiving or have developed a tolerance to pain therapy with products known as opioids. Duragesic should not be used if you have pain that will go away in a few days, such as pain from surgery, medical or dental procedures, or short-lasting conditions."

Fentanyl, the medication in the patch, takes six to twelve hours or more to reach a therapeutic level in the bloodstream. It also takes many hours for it to leave the bloodstream after the patch is removed. If your dog has side effects (and there are many), removing the patch will not alleviate his discomfort or illness for hours. You may not even know he is having side effects. Common side effects include somnolence and confusion, which in a dog could easily be mistaken for well-managed pain.

In 2014, a medication was approved by the FDA for post-op pain in dogs. It is called Recuvyra®, and the drug is fentanyl. The drug is delivered through a specially designed applicator rather than a patch, and released onto the skin. The manufacturer warns that no children or other pets should come into contact with the application site for three full days. This is basically the same as the "pain patch," but without the patch.

Recuvyra is available from Elanco™. An April 2014 article posted at www.DVM360.com bears the headline, "Eli Lilly to buy Novartis Animal Health, merge assets with Elanco. $5.4 billion deal to create one of the world's largest veterinary health companies." Draw your own conclusions. I would not allow the Duragesic patch or Recuvyra to be used on my dog for post-operative pain.

Similarly, the drug Neurontin® (gabapentin) became very popular among veterinarians for post-operative pain in the early 2000s. It was originally approved and released for human use as an anti-seizure medication. Later, it was found to be effective for chronic neurogenic pain. Like the fentanyl patch, this drug's pharmaceutical insert states emphatically that it should be used for chronic pain only, not for acute short-term pain, and never for post-surgery pain.

I would not give this medication to my dog unless he had seizures or chronic nerve pain. I do not believe it should be prescribed for a dog (or person) to treat post-surgery pain. Just as I stated above regarding the fentanyl patch, common side effects of gabapentin include somnolence and confusion, which in a dog could be mistaken for well-managed pain.

6

Radiation Therapy for Canine Cancer

R adiation therapy works by damaging the DNA in cancer cells, so the cells cannot replicate and create new cancer cells. When any tumor can be entirely and safely removed, surgery with wide margins is always preferable to radiation therapy (RTx), and carries a much more optimistic prognosis. RTx is a distant second choice. The most predictable benefit of RTx is not to cure cancer, but to stop bleeding, relieve pressure, alleviate pain, shrink a tumor, and possibly slow down the progression of cancer.

RTx is most effective before surgery, to shrink a tumor and improve the potential success of the surgery. It is possible for controlled doses of radiation to reduce the size of a tumor. Once the tumor has been made smaller, particularly if it is near bone or muscle tissue, the surgeon has a better chance of being able to remove it entirely with wide margins and without cutting into bone or muscle tissue. This use of RTx is only preparatory. The success of the dog's treatment will depend on the surgery results.

When surgery is not an option, RTx is often used to treat tumors in the brain, nasal cavity, or mouth. A soft-tissue tumor, such as a mast cell or melanoma tumor, may be treated with radiation therapy if the tumor has not metastasized and cannot be surgically removed. It is not effective against a cancer that has metastasized. When RTx is given for a tumor that has not been surgically removed, the possible benefits are palliative.

RTx can be given to a dog with cancer in a leg (usually bone cancer) as an alternative to amputation for dogs that are not candidates for amputation. A dog may not be a candidate for amputation due to age or other health issues (such as lameness or weakness in another leg). In many cases, a dog may not be a candidate only because the owner is not willing or emotionally able to agree to amputation surgery.

In lieu of amputation, radiation therapy is usually used in conjunction with limb-sparing surgery. When the dog has osteosarcoma, this treatment option avoids amputation but does not extend survival times significantly. For the owner, limb sparing is less traumatic than amputation for the owner, but may be more difficult and more painful for the dog.

▷ *Lacy Jenkins' Story*

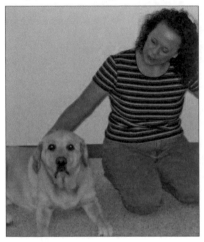

My husband and I were truly blessed that Lacy was part of our family for nine years. Lacy loved everyone and everyone loved her.

When Lacy was nine, I noticed that she was limping and had a slight swelling on one of her rear legs. Our veterinarian performed a biopsy and said that Lacy had cancer.

The word cancer sent fear piercing through our veins. The good news, he said, was that the cancer had not spread and was contained in the soft tissue of her leg rather than the bone.

Amputation was one treatment option and the alternative was surgery to remove the tumor, followed by a series of radiation therapy treatments to prevent the tumor from returning. We decided as a family that we were not prepared for an amputation as long as there was another option.

There was hope for Lacy's long term survival, but it would cost more than we could afford. I have done animal rescue and fostered many animals, but now that my own dog needed help our family was financially strapped. So I searched for help. I found the Magic Bullet Fund and they agreed to help us.

We started making Bullet's Cancer Diet for Lacy and giving her supplements, to strengthen her immune system and help her fight cancer.

On February 23, 2007, Dr. Joe Hendricks removed Lacy's tumor and was elated about the result. Then, to our surprise, he referred us to radiation oncologist Dr. Joyce Obradovich for eighteen treatments of radiation therapy over three and a half weeks.

Dr. Obradovich said that Lacy's prognosis was very good. Sadly, Lacy passed in June of 2007.

Ronda Jenkins, Grand Blanc, Michigan

When a dog is going to have traditional radiation therapy, called "external beam radiation," the treatment plan is created in reference to a total dose needed, and the total dose is divided into fractions. At each treatment, one fraction is delivered.

Radiation therapy does not predictably "cure cancer." How can I say this when there are radiation protocols that are called "curative?" Veterinarians often ask an owner to choose between "curative radiation" and "palliative radiation" protocols. These two terms are misnomers. They make the owner feel as though he needs to decide: "Do you want to give your dog a chance to survive cancer, or just give him a little more time?"

The low-dose protocol, even though it is called "palliative," often turns out to be curative! Sometimes the cancer does not return. The high-dose protocol, even though it is called "curative," often does not get rid of the cancer or prevent it from returning. Let's instead call these protocols "high-dose" and "low-dose" radiation.

High-dose radiation therapy for dogs generally means treatment every day, Monday through Friday. Often the dog ends up with skin burns that may become infected and may never heal. Sometimes, the dog dies during a curative radiation protocol. Sometimes the clinic wants the dog to stay at the clinic Monday through Friday and go home on weekends. This separation is hard on the dogs and hard on the owners.

Low-dose radiation protocols may call for three treatments a week for nine, fifteen or eighteen treatments, or once a week for four to twelve weeks. Low-dose protocols are easier on the dog and on the owner. The dog goes home every night, side effects are mild if present at all, and it is much less expensive.

Low-dose RTx can be used post-surgically if a tumor was not completely removed. The radiation is given not to cure the cancer but to shrink the tumor, make the dog more comfortable and possibly to provide longer survival. If the tumor is expected to return aggressively after surgery, some additional time may be gained by radiation treatments.

Many tumors that remain after surgery will be nonaggressive, slow-growing, and will not metastasize for many months or more than a year. The grade of a cancer is a useful tool in predicting whether or not an incompletely removed cancer will be aggressive and grow quickly.

The owner must decide whether the possibility of gaining a few extra weeks or months justifies the trauma to their dog and the expense to them. Join a canine cancer group that has the largest member list. Ask the group questions to find out how long dogs with the type of cancer your dog has, and with similar surgical results, survived when given radiation. Then ask how long dogs with the same cancer and similar surgical results survived who were not given radiation treatments.

A dog may have successful surgery followed by radiation treatment because the biopsy report stated: "microscopic disease may remain." The dog may survive many years. Did the dog survive because of the radiation treatments? Or did the dog survive because after the surgery there was no microscopic disease remaining?

Learning that "microscopic disease may remain," a dog's owner may feel panicked and say "that is terrible, we must get rid of all of the cancer cells!" As stated earlier, I believe that the phrase should be replaced by: "Microscopic disease may or may not remain." Pathologists would be hard pressed to ever guarantee that all cancer cells have been killed off and the tumor will not return. They need to err on the side of caution.

When the biopsy report after surgery shows clean but narrow margins and a possibility of "microscopic disease," you can leave it alone, or you can put your dog through further treatment. In case stray cancers cells actually do remain and your dog's immune system cannot fight them, you may feel compelled to provide additional treatment. Low-dose radiation therapy is an option, but be aware that additional treatment (radiation therapy or chemotherapy) may get rid of the cells that may remain, or it may not.

It is your choice whether to provide a high-dose or low-dose radiation protocol for your dog's cancer. In fact, it is your choice whether to provide radiation therapy at all. Don't be swayed by peer pressure or by your veterinarian. Your vet should support your decision. If your veterinarian objects to your choice, find a new veterinarian. For some vets, an opportunity to provide treatment is more important than your dog's quality of life.

▷ ***Nakkai Driber's Story***

   Nakkai had surgery to remove a nerve sheath tumor (schwannoma) in her leg. Nakkai's surgeon, Dr. Dundas, told me that he would probably not be able to remove the entire tumor. He recommended amputation but Sharon refused.

   The surgeon was very surprised and excited. He said to me on the phone that the entire tumor lifted out in one piece, and Nakkai may not need radiation therapy at all.

   The biopsy report stated that the margins were narrow at best.

   Nakkai's radiation oncologist, Dr. Looper at VCA Aurora Animal Hospital, said that Nakkai should have a curative course of radiation therapy. She presented one option. It was the standard radiation protocol that most veterinary radiation oncologists recommend for the dogs, and it calls for a treatment once a day, Monday through Friday, for four weeks. Nakkai would stay at the clinic during the week and go home on weekends.

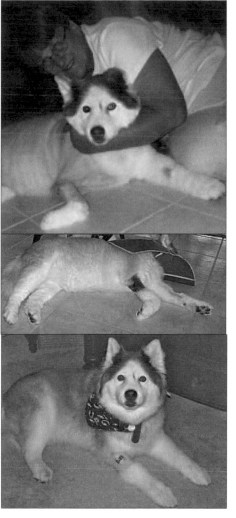

   Nakkai's mom, Sharon, agreed to let me request a less aggressive, less traumatic, and less expensive protocol for Nakkai. I requested a three-day-a-week protocol. Nakkai would have treatments Monday, Wednesday, and Friday for four weeks and would go home after each treatment.

*The veterinarian said that she couldn't give Nakkai a less aggres-
sive protocol. She said she couldn't even find one to use. When
treatment day came and neither I nor the owner had signed the treatment plan, Dr. Looper called me to say she had found a "palliative"
protocol to use after all. We all agreed to the three-day per week
protocol for Nakkai.*

*Nakkai had minimal side effects—only a radiation burn at the
surgery site. The open sore healed in about a month, but the skin
remained black, and the hair did not grow back. Sharon protected the
skin with jazzy sports wristbands.*

*Nakkai was diagnosed in June 2007 and survived with great
quality of life until November 27, 2011. The cancer never returned. As
it turned out, the "palliative" protocol for Nakkai was "curative."*

- Laurie Kaplan

Other types of radiation treatment available for dogs with cancer:

Intraoperative Radiation

One external beam treatment is given after surgery, directly into the
surgery site, to discourage recurrence. I have not found any studies that
compare surgery success with and without intraoperative radiation.

Stereotactic Radiosurgery

This includes CyberKnife® and gamma knife treatments. These tools
offer thin slits of highly focused beams of radiation and are used most
often for inoperable tumors in the brain or the pituitary gland. They can be
used in a single treatment for tumors smaller than 1 inch in diameter. For
larger tumors, they can be used in several treatments (fractionated stereotactic radiotherapy).

For the following, dog is in isolation until radioactivity is expelled.

Brachytherapy

Radioactive implants are placed into the surgical site after the tumor is
removed. If surgery is not an option, the implants are placed directly into
the tumor. This is often used for nasal tumors.

Radioactive Iodine Therapy

This treatment is given for thyroid cancer. Radioiodine (I-131) is injected. When it enters the thyroid gland, it destroys the cancer cells.

Radioisotope (systemic) Radiation

A radioactive isotope is given orally or by injection. The isotope is known to be absorbed specifically by the organ tissue or the tumor.

Radioimmunotherapy

This combines a monoclonal antibody, such as Zevalin®, with a radioisotope. This is given by an intravenous infusion and is often used to treat leukemia.

Intensity-Modulated Radiation Therapy (IMRT)

IMRT is a method of delivering radiation to a tumor while shaping the radiation beams to the shape of the tumor. This can allow the use of high doses of radiation while reducing side effects by minimizing the amount of radiation that is unintentionally delivered to your dog's healthy tissues. IMRT may be used in stereotactic radiation or stereotactic radiation.

7

Chemotherapy
for Canine Cancer

C ancer is the "C word" that makes us cringe most, but chemotherapy is a close runner-up. Chemotherapy is used to treat many canine cancers, including lymphoma, leukemia, multiple myeloma, systemic mast cell, soft-tissue sarcoma, osteosarcoma, and carcinoma.

Some dog owners are against putting their dog through chemotherapy. They may have seen a friend undergo chemotherapy only to become deathly ill. They may have a family member who died in spite of, or because of, chemotherapy.

Dogs tolerate chemotherapy better than people do. Chemotherapy protocols for dogs are less aggressive than those designed for humans. The dogs get a kinder, gentler version of the treatments that are given to people, and the recommended dosages are lower. While people may be willing to undergo extreme, potentially life-threatening treatment in order to have a chance at beating cancer or to survive a few extra months, most pet owners are not willing to see their dogs die or become severely ill from treatment.

In veterinary oncology, the recommended dosages of chemo drugs are those that will make only 10 percent or less of the dogs have serious side effects. For dogs that have side effects, pre-treating with antihistamines, such as Benadryl, can be helpful.

The most common side effects are nausea (which can begin soon after treatment), and diarrhea (which usually sets in five to seven days after a treatment). See the Side Effects chapter for help dealing with these and other side effects. Speak to your vet about all side effects your dog has. If any of them become severe, talk to your vet about lowering the dosages of the chemo drugs.

People in chemotherapy lose their hair. Our hair is constantly growing, and therefore the hair cells are constantly dividing. Most dogs renew their coats seasonally, and so they usually do not experience hair loss from chemotherapy. The dogs that are most likely to lose hair are those that are considered hypoallergenic dogs, and have a coat that is hair-like rather than fur-like.

Some dogs have a hard time with chemotherapy. Aggressive dogs must be restrained or muzzled. Fearful dogs shake and become distressed. Multi-drug chemotherapy protocols using IV treatments are not the best choice for a dog that would be traumatized by weekly treatments. They may need to be anesthetized for each treatment. If this is the case, ask your vet about chemo treatments that you can give your dog at home, in pill form.

Any dog might be stressed during the first chemotherapy treatment. It is a new experience. They do not know what is being done to them. Don't give up right away. Some dogs get used to the procedure and become more relaxed with subsequent treatments.

Bullet was decidedly not the model patient during his first few chemotherapy sessions. During the first treatment, Dr. Porzio came out to the waiting room to tell me with his adorable Italian accent, "The Bullet is very strong!" Apparently, he had thrown the good veterinarian across the room. Bullet cried, squirmed, and growled. He nipped Rod, the fellow whose job it was to get him to lay still.

But after the first few treatments, Bullet did become the model patient. Dr. Porzio often emerged from a treatment saying that Bullet had been "an angel." He stayed still, quiet, and comfortable, and gave kisses to staff members holding him—especially Rod! Bullet demonstrated that dogs can adapt and become more agreeable to treatment in a short time.

Traditional Chemotherapy

Like all cancer treatment, chemotherapy is a balancing act. High dosages give a better chance of killing the cancer, and a higher chance of producing side effects. Low dosages may sidestep side effects, but may not be strong enough to kill the cancer. Dosages can and should be adjusted and customized to suit the dog. Make sure your vet knows your feelings about how aggressively you want to fight your dog's cancer.

Express Your Wishes

▸ You can request the strongest treatment, which may have the best chance of killing the cancer but also carries a higher probability of severe side effects, up to and including death.

▸ You can request a gentler treatment plan that may have a lower chance of killing the cancer but also reduces the chance that your dog will become ill from side effects.

▸ You can decide that you want your dog to receive the standard protocol with middle-range dosages, and be prepared to adjust dosages according to the cancer's response to treatment.

If your dog needs chemotherapy, participate in choosing the chemotherapy protocol that should be used, and how aggressively it should be used. Ask your veterinarian to provide you with a treatment plan for your dog's chemotherapy protocol. The plan should show which drug will be given at each treatment, and how many weeks there are between treatments. Request an estimated fee for each treatment on the list. (See Most Common Protocols in Appendix.)

Other Decisions You Can Make

▸ Leave or wait? If being left at the veterinarian's office is stressful for your dog, sit with him in the waiting room until they are ready to give him treatment, and take him home when the treatment is finished. No one wants to be in a hospital longer than necessary—dogs included. A dog should never have to stay in the clinic overnight for a chemotherapy treatment unless something goes wrong.

▸ Shaving: It's easy to wind up with a patchwork dog, so keep the shaving to a minimum from the start. It's necessary to shave some fur before surgery or chemotherapy. Ask your vet to shave a little as possible. It's usually not necessary to shave fur for a blood test. With a little extra effort, a vet can draw blood without shaving. Make an effort to preserve the beauty and natural integrity of the animal. Keep your dog intact and beautiful during treatment.

▶ Which leg? You can specify which leg should be used for testing and treatment. If, for example, your dog is favoring a leg for any reason, request that a different leg be used for treatment.

When Bullet's chemotherapy started, Dr. Porzio had difficulty finding a vein in which to insert the catheter. Through this catheter, the chemotherapy agent would be delivered. When Bullet emerged, he had a shaved square on each of his four limbs.

For an entire year, I asked Dr. Porzio to continue to use the vein in Bullet's left rear leg, re-shaving the same patch when necessary and allowing the fur to grow in over the other patches. I anticipated that, at some point, Dr. Porzio would tell me that the vein was no longer usable, and we'd have to switch to another leg.

After the first year of treatment, I asked Dr. Porzio to switch to the right rear leg and give the left rear vein a rest. I had a feeling the vein that was used repeatedly for so long would collapse.

About Chemotherapy

Chemotherapy is the administration of one or more agents (drugs) designed to kill cancer cells, or at least hinder their ability to multiply and progress. The most significant behavior that makes cancer cells different from healthy cells is that they undergo cell division much more frequently.

The objective, therefore, is to use chemo agents that will attack cells that are dividing. Each agent attacks cells in a specific phase of cell division. Chemotherapy kills many cancer cells during a treatment, as well as some innocent, healthy cells that happen to be dividing.

Some chemo agents are given intravenously, some are injected subcutaneously, and some are given in pill form. Intravenous treatments are generally given through a catheter, and setting up the delivery system can take time.

Treatment duration for IV chemotherapy varies depending on the size of the dog. Dosages are calculated according to the body surface area (BSA) of the dog, which can be roughly translated into weight. The larger the dog, the greater the volume of chemotherapy agent that must be given. An infusion for a large dog takes longer especially for an infusion.

Doxorubicin (Adriamycin, or Adria) is not simply injected into the vein.

It is more effective and less likely to produce cardiotoxic side effects when given as an infusion or a drip.

However, the longer the infusion, the greater the risk for extravasation. The catheterization site should be watched very carefully during the entire infusion because of the possibility of extravasation. Generally, infusions are given for twenty minutes to two hours.

▷ **Tensing Summers' Story**

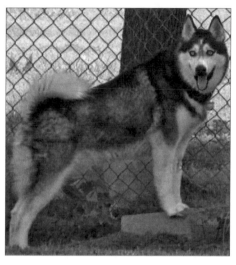

Tensing was Karen's beloved Siberian husky. He had lymphoma and started chemo in February of 2007. His veterinarian had treated only a handful of canine cancer patients but there were no veterinary oncologists in this rural area. The veterinarian was providing a needed service to but she was not well informed about the basics of administering chemotherapy for dogs.

After a four treatments, Dr. B. told Karen that Tensing was in remission, and that therefore he did not need to continue chemotherapy. Tensing came out of remission in three weeks. In April 2008, Tensing came into the Magic Bullet Fund and chemotherapy was restarted.

When the invoice for Tensing's treatment showed charges for an overnight stay at the clinic, I called Karen to ask why he was there overnight. She said that Tensing was kept overnight for every chemo treatment. I called the clinic to ask why, and was told that Tensing had eighteen-hour chemotherapy infusions, left in a clinic kennel unattended through the night. Tensing was extremely lucky that an extravasation did not occur!

Dr. B. agreed to limit the infusions to not more than one hour. With these problems straightened out, Tensing's treatment continued properly and he remained in remission until December 2008. This was *a successful fight against cancer. Tensing went to the Rainbow Bridge on December 15, 2008, twenty-two months after his diagnosis, at nine years old.*

- Laurie Kaplan

Some veterinarians test cardiac functions before giving a dog the first Adria treatment, but not before subsequent treatments unless the dog shows signs of cardiac problems.

Some vets want to run cardiac tests before every treatment with Adria, and others do not run cardiac tests at all, unless the dog has a history of cardiac problems or is a breed that is predisposed to cardiac problems. Cardiac tests may include electro cardiogram, x-ray and/or ultrasound.

When finances are tight and the dog has no known heart problems, owners have the option of bypassing the cardiac tests, as long as their dog hasn't had an amount of Adria approaching the maximum lifetime dosage for the dog's body surface area. This amount is generally five treatments at the recommended dosages.

Some veterinarians prefer to give chemotherapy treatment to a fasted dog. If your vet has no objections, encourage your dog to drink water before IV chemotherapy treatment. This will to dilate his veins and make the insertion of a catheter simpler for the veterinarian and less traumatic for your dog.

About Chemotherapy Protocols

A chemotherapy *protocol* is an attack plan. It specifies which chemotherapy drugs (agents) will be given, in what order, and the dosages and schedule by which they will be given, week by week, from beginning to end. You can find examples of the most common chemotherapy protocols used for dogs with cancer in the Appendix.

When there is more than one protocol that might help, choosing which protocol to use is a strategic decision, similar to deciding whether to deploy the marines, the air force, or the navy to attack an enemy.

Different protocols are used for different types of cancer, and usually there is more than one viable protocol for any particular type of cancer. Each protocol is unique in terms of which agents it includes, in what order, and on what schedule.

Keep track of your dog's treatments. You should always know what treatment will be given next, which drug, and how much it will cost. Ask your vet to give you a printout showing the protocol he is using to treat your dog.

A high percentage of the chemotherapy treatments given to dogs with cancer are given to dogs with lymphoma. In the following text, I often use lymphoma as an example, although the same principles apply for other cancers treated with chemotherapy.

There are single-agent protocols, which use one agent repeatedly until the patient comes out of remission, and there are combination protocols. Single-agent protocols are used for cancers such as osteosarcoma and transitional cell carcinoma. In the past, a single-agent Adriamycin protocol was used regularly for lymphoma. Some oncologists still use it, but combination protocols are generally considered to be more effective against lymphoma.

In a combination chemotherapy protocol, each agent attacks cancer in a different way (i.e., at a different stage during the replication of the cell). Agents are given in rotation according to a schedule, to attack cancer cells with one drug, then another, then another.

The theory behind a combination protocol is that no one chemotherapy agent will consistently and reliably "cure" cancer. Unfortunately, there is no "Magic Bullet," except the one who used to snooze in my living room. For this reason, chemotherapy protocols often include several drugs and they are given in rotation.

Each agent used in a course of chemotherapy is effective to some degree, alone or in combination with other agents. Most chemo agents attack cells that are dividing, but some agents, such as L-asparaginase (L-Spar), behave differently. L-Spar weakens dividing cells so that the next chemo agent, given within a week, can kill those cells more effectively. An L-Spar treatment should be followed about a week later by a treatment with another agent.

The name of a protocol is often an acronym, using the first letter of each drug. Most protocols include prednisone, thus the final "P" in the protocol names. The VELCAP protocol includes the agents vincristine, Elspar, Cytoxan, Adriamycin, and prednisone. The most widely used protocol for canine lymphoma is the Modified Madison-Wisconsin

Protocol, which also includes these same four agents. Other protocols are named CHOP, COP, CLOP, and MOPP. The "O" in these protocols is Oncovin®, a brand name for vincristine.

When the owner is willing and the dog tolerates treatment, a chemotherapy protocol is given until its end, as long as the dog stays in remission. If the dog comes out of remission, the lymph nodes become enlarged again. When remission is lost sometime later, and the cancer is active, then chemotherapy can begin again in an attempt to achieve a second remission.

A second remission is more difficult to achieve. Only about 40 percent of dogs achieve a second remission. In general, the second remission lasts about half as long as the first, and each subsequent remission lasts a shorter time. A dog can go in and out of remission five times or more.

When a dog comes out of remission before the first chemotherapy protocol has been completed, the veterinarian will switch to a different protocol using different chemo drugs. Clearly the drugs in use were not successful. One study notes that the failure of one chemotherapy protocol to keep a dog in remission can be seen as a predictor that chemotherapy is simply not going to be able to control that particular cancer in that particular dog. The study, titled "Relative Mitochondrial Priming of Myeloblasts and Normal HSCs Determines Chemotherapeutic Success in AML" was published in *Cell Press*, October 2012.

When a dog comes out of remission after a protocol has been completed, a decision must be made. The same protocol may be given again in hopes of another remission, or a different protocol may be used.

If your dog does not go into remission using the standard protocol, or suffers intolerable side effects, then there is a reason to improvise or switch to another protocol.

L-Spar is often very effective in gaining a remission. The Modified Madison-Wisconsin Protocol, as given in the late 1900s and early 2000s, included L-Spar as the first treatment. However, a recent study at the University of Wisconsin-Madison found that the success of the protocol is the same whether or not L-Spar is given at the first treatment. The conclusion was that while L-Spar is a powerful agent in gaining a remission, it may prove to be more effective for long term survival if it is withheld until a dog comes out of remission.

A commonly used rescue protocol is CCNU (lomustine) with prednisone. Some veterinarians recommend using L-Spar with CCNU as a rescue protocol, particularly if it has not been used in the first protocol. Yet another study found that using L-Spar with CCNU does not afford a longer survival time, and may cause toxicity.

Select a Protocol

It may be tempting to agree to any and all treatments your veterinarian offers. Before you agree to give your dog anything other than the standard treatment, ask your vet to show you proof that the treatment is at least as successful as the standard treatment. Ask for an article in a veterinary journal describing the trial. How many dogs were included in the study? Did dogs survive longer than they would have with a standard protocol?

Trials and studies are always underway concerning cancer treatments for dogs. They each present a potentially useful theory, but most employ a very small study group. When the number of dogs is less than 1,000, studies and trials should not necessarily be seen as evidence that a treatment will be successful. The conclusions may or may not hold true in a larger study group.

Many veterinary oncologists are involved in clinical trials that use the standard array of drugs in different combinations, on different treatment schedules, or with different dosages. Some devise their own personal variation of a protocol and prefer to administer their version of the protocol to their canine cancer patients. Their way may or may not prove to have a better success rate than the standard protocol.

One owner applied to the Magic Bullet Fund for her dog's treatment. Her dog had lymphoma, and the veterinary oncologist emailed me a protocol that was very unusual. It was complicated, convoluted, included seven different chemo drugs to be given in what looked like a haphazard order and combinations. It looked as though it would promise severe side effects, and it was very expensive. It looked like a CHOP protocol, CCNU protocol and MOPP protocol all jumbled together.

I asked the vet if she used this protocol for all of her canine lymphoma patients. She said, "No, only those who can afford it." I found this very amusing, since she knew the owner had applied to the Magic Bullet Fund for financial assistance.

I sent the protocol to a veterinary oncologist friend, asking for their opinion and to find out if they recognized the protocol. She responded, "What is the name of the oncologist that is parading this pricey interposed protocol? It's no surprise that the dogs had more neutropenia! I wonder how many had grade IV adverse events and toxicity?"

With a little research I discovered that the veterinarian had been involved in a clinical trial for a new chemo protocol for lymphoma. The protocol had failed to produce better survival rates, but the veterinarian was still administering it to her patients.

This vet may be finding it difficult to give up on the protocol. She put her time, energy and hopes into developing a new protocol and cannot give it up, even when studies show lack of success. Perhaps she was still making a effort to get long survival rates using the protocol.

I know of several cases (and surely there are many more) where a veterinarian recommends an unproven protocol to use (i.e., test) on a client's dog. They say to the client that this protocol should be given to your dog because it will give him the best chance of survival.

When a trusted veterinarian recommends a procedure, the owner often consents without knowing much about it. An ethical veterinarian always tells clients what is known about the efficacy or proven success rate of a proposed treatment plan, and will always tell the client if a drug or a treatment is experimental.

How Much is Enough?

It's a tricky business trying to determine how much treatment is needed to eradicate the cancer without eradicating the dog. Too little treatment will not kill the cancer. Too much treatment may kill the patient.

The objective of a chemo protocol is to provide the type, amount, strength, and frequency of treatments that will eradicate the cancer cells without doing irreparable damage to healthy cells. The duration of a protocol is determined by studies that help to find the point of diminishing return. That is the point beyond which the survival time is not expected to increase if more chemotherapy treatments are given. Let's say one hundred dogs are tested, and the average survival time is the same for the fifty dogs who receive sixteen treatments as it is for the fifty dogs that receive thirty-two treatments. Since the additional sixteen treatments did not result in longer survival, this study would conclude that there is no benefit to giving the final sixteen treatments, and the protocol would be shortened to a total of sixteen treatments.

Bullet's protocol in 2000 ran for seventy-five weeks. In the early 2000s, a study showed that overall survival time was the same whether a dog had the long VELCAP-L protocol (hoping for a long remission), or a short twenty-six-week version (VELCAP-S), followed by more chemotherapy, if and when he came out of remission.

When chemotherapy protocols for dogs became shorter in the early 2000s, I asked Dr. Cotter for an explanation, and she offered the following (email, 9/9/2013):

> *"Most dogs—particularly those with B-cell lymphoma as opposed to T-cell—don't require eighteen months of chemotherapy." Protocols that run for nineteen to twenty-six weeks, such as the very popular Modified Madison-Wisconsin protocol or another CHOP protocol, became the gold standard for canine lymphoma treatment. These protocols spare a dog from having more chemotherapy than is needed and have a fee structure that more dog owners are able to afford."*

You may begin to feel apprehensive when your dog's chemo protocol is nearing the end. It is very common for an owner to think, *"Treatment is keeping my dog's cancer away. When chemotherapy stops the cancer will return."* Sometime around 2008, perhaps to assuage these fears or perhaps to exploit them, "maintenance chemotherapy" became popular. Before that time, a dog finished a protocol and the treatments ended. In maintenance chemotherapy, additional treatments are tacked onto the end of a protocol. I call them "forever protocols."

Studies show that survival times are the same whether treatment stops at the end of the protocol (if cancer returns, more chemo is given), or treatments are continued indefinitely. The Merck Veterinary Manual says:

> *"A discontinuous chemotherapy protocol is used more commonly in veterinary oncology than maintenance or continuous chemotherapy.*

Discontinuous chemotherapy in dogs appears to lead to the same or similar remission and survival time as a traditional maintenance protocol. In this approach, all chemotherapy is discontinued for patients that are in complete remission at the end of the treatment protocol. At the first signs of recurrence of lymphoma, reinduction using the original chemotherapy protocol should be used. Studies have suggested that dogs receiving a discontinuous protocol were more likely to achieve a second remission when they relapsed than dogs that received long term or maintenance chemotherapy. If reinduction fails, use of rescue protocols should be considered."

An article published in the *Journal of Veterinary Internal Medicine*, November 2002, titled "Evaluation of a 6-Month Chemotherapy Protocol With no Maintenance Therapy for Dogs with Lymphoma," states, "The six-month chemotherapy protocol based on CHOP with no maintenance phase provides similar … survival times when compared to a similar protocol with a prolonged maintenance phase." In other words, nothing is gained by continuing chemotherapy.

Overtreatment

There are good reasons not to provide more treatment than is necessary and curative. Ideally, you want to give enough to kill the cancer but not one drop more. If and when the dog comes out of remission, more treatment can be given.

Additional treatments put a dog at risk for extravasation, neuropathy, anaphylaxis, organ damage, myelosuppression or death. Dogs can become lame from chemotherapy treatments, develop hemorrhagic cystitis of the bladder, or cardiomyopathy and heart failure. Most chemo drugs can damage the bone marrow. All chemotherapy drugs damage cells. That is how they kill cancer.

Not to mention that continued treatments and trips to the clinic must have a negative effect on a dog's quality of life. Not to mention that continued treatment has a negative effect on the owner's bank account.

Giving a dog more chemotherapy than necessary is one type of overtreatment. When the standard treatment is not working, and a second-line protocol is not working, there are still other chemo drugs to try. Should you try them all on the off chance that one might work? We want so desperately to help our dogs fight cancer and survive. We might be tempted to try them all.

There should be a point in time when we stop throwing endless treatments at a dog's cancer when the treatments are not effective. These dogs should be allowed to enjoy survival as long as there is good quality of life without receiving shot-in-the-dark treatments that have little or no hope of success, but will surely diminish their quality of life in their last days, weeks, or months. The dog's quality of life and the family's opportunity to prepare for a loss should be important. At some point, the veterinarian's job is not to cheer the owner on with false hope, but to help the owner accept that treatment is not working.

The veterinary community seems to have forgotten about palliative care. Palliative care means hospice, pawspice, or end-of-life care. In palliative care, you do not aim to cure or fight your dog's cancer. You maximize his comfort level and quality of life during the time he has left, and you hope to prolong that period of time.

If a vet encourages more treatment after treatments have failed, in the best light we can say that he is working so hard to save the dog that he refuses to give up. Sometimes the owner has to be the one to say it is time to provide palliative care.

A parallel can be seen between overtreatment in veterinary medicine and overtreatment in human medicine. Shannon Brownlee, author of *Overtreated: Why Too Much Medicine Is Making Us Sicker and Poorer*, writes about human medicine, "An epidemic of overtreatment—too many scans, too many blood tests, too many procedures—is costing the nation's health care system at least $210 billion a year, according to the Institute of Medicine, and taking a human toll in pain, emotional suffering, severe complications, and even death."

Undertreatment

What is undertreatment? In surgery, undertreatment can mean not excising a tumor that could be removed, or not removing enough tissue around a tumor. Removing excess healthy tissue around the tumor is better than not removing enough, as long as no bone or muscle tissue is removed unnecessarily.

In chemo and radiation therapy, if the protocol is not completed, the treatment may help the dog but there will be a smaller chance of long term survival than when recommended dosages and treatments are given.

I did say earlier that you can begin treatment and then stop at any point, that there is no contract saying you have to give all of the treatments. If there are financial constraints, however, or if the dog's health is precarious, giving some treatment is better than giving none. When given half of a protocol for lymphoma for example, most dogs will go into remission but will not stay in remission as long as if the protocol is completed.

When remission is achieved, this does not mean that chemotherapy ends. It is common knowledge that our doctors prescribe antibiotics, the entire prescription should be taken even if we are feeling better halfway through. Similarly, the entire chemotherapy protocol for our dogs should be completed even after remission has been achieved. Failure to complete the protocol may be seen as undertreatment.

Hopefully chemotherapy will put cancer into remission, but remission is only the first step. Most dogs with lymphoma, for example, go into remission after the first one or two treatments. But if chemotherapy stops at that point, the cancer will return quickly.

If a dog's owner chooses to end treatment before the final treatments, the dog might stay in remission. However, if the dog relapses and dies, the owner would probably regret this decision and always wonder if how long his dog would have survived if the protocol had been completed.

A better decision is to give the final treatments, but discount (lower the dosages of) the drugs by 15 to 20 percent. This will minimize side effects, and lower the fees as well. Or, give treatments on a looser schedule (every three weeks instead of every two weeks). Or you can do both.

Intralesional Chemotherapy

Chemotherapy drugs are usually given intravenously, by injection, or as a pill. They can also be injected directly into a tumor or into a site where a tumor or part of a tumor has been removed. With intralesional chemotherapy, the tumor and stray cancer cells receive a much greater dose of the drug than they do via intravenous chemotherapy. The drug is given without any need for it to circulate through the body.

There is collateral damage to healthy cells, since the injected drug spreads. It is intended to spread to kill healthy cells outside of the tumor, so that stray cancer cells and microscopic disease can be attacked. In intralesional chemo, the collateral damage occurs locally rather than throughout the entire body.

The same side effects are seen as with IV chemo. Studies are under way to establish dosages for intralesional chemotherapy that will yield a high cancer cell kill rate and the lowest side effects possible.

This method of chemotherapy is being analyzed for various types of tumors, including soft tissue sarcoma, osteosarcoma, squamous cell carcinoma, and oral malignant melanoma. Studies and trials for intralesional chemotherapy use various chemo drugs, including carboplatin, mitoxantrone, cisplatin, and bleomycin.

Electrochemotherapy

In the early 1990s, research studies were published exploring the anti-tumor effect of using chemotherapy plus electrical pulses to treat solid tumors. This method is used with chemotherapy drugs that are unable to cross a cell membrane, such as bleomycin or cisplatin.

The chemotherapy drug is delivered to the tumor. Shortly afterward, electrical pulses are delivered directly to the tumor via electrodes. Theoretically, the pulses enable the drugs to cross the cell membranes and attack the cancer cells.

Electrochemotherapy can be used intraoperatively for inoperable solid tumors as well as for cutaneous and subcutaneous tumors.

Medical Cautions

Anyone who has a dog receiving chemotherapy should be aware of the potential consequences of treatment. These are medical hazards, not to be confused with the side effects as discussed in the next chapter. These conditions are very serious and cannot be remedied at home.

Myelosuppression

One thing that is known about cancer cells is that they divide (replicate) more frequently than most healthy cells. For this reason, chemotherapy drugs are designed to fight cancer by targeting cells that are in the process of dividing. They don't target cancer cells specifically. They target any cells that are dividing.

Stem cells in the bone marrow are responsible for producing new blood cells. They produce red and white blood cells and platelets, which are all necessary for survival. Bone marrow cells divide more frequently than other healthy cells in the body, and are therefore at high risk for being attacked by chemotherapy drugs.

The most serious side effect of chemotherapy is *myelosuppression*. The bone marrow's ability to produce new blood cells is crippled. Some degree of myelosuppression is expected after chemotherapy because the chemo drugs attack the cells in the bone marrow as well as the cancer cells.

It's not unusual for a dog's white blood count (WBC) and neutrophils to plummet a week to ten days after a treatment. With a low WBC, a dog might feel crappy and be lethargic.

A complete blood count (CBC) is done before each treatment, to ensure that the WBC is not too low (due to the previous treatment) to give treatment. If it is too low, the veterinarian will postpone the treatment. Cutoff points vary from veterinarian to veterinarian, but a white blood cell count lower than about 3,000 and/or neutrophil count lower than about 2,000 usually prompts a one-week postponement. Usually, the white count recovers in one week and then treatment continues.

If the WBC drops below 1,000 this is *neutropenia*—an emergency situation that must be treated quickly by a veterinarian. Neutropenia is accompanied by a high fever, so take your dog's temperature every few days after a chemo treatment if you can. You might discover neutropenia early, so your vet can provide treatment right away.

Your vet may provide antibiotics to prevent infection while your dog is immunosuppressed. He may prescribe Neupogen® (filgrastim) to increase the number of neutrophils in the blood.

When chemotherapy has to be postponed more than once due to a low WBC (lower than 3,000), or when chemotherapy causes neutropenia even once, the chemo protocol should be revised.

Fighting cancer is a balancing act.
The challenge is to find the treatment that is strong enough
to kill the cancer but not strong enough to kill the patient.

The amount of pain medication that I need after a surgery is different from the amount that you need after the same surgery. Dogs also have different reactions and tolerances to drugs, including chemotherapy drugs.

To revise a protocol, your vet can lower the dose of the chemo agent. It may make sense to lower dosages of all of the drugs, or only of the one that caused the myelosuppression. Discuss this with your vet. Another option is to exclude the drug that caused the myelosuppression from the rest of the protocol and replace it with a different drug.

Extravasation

Extravasation (translated "outside of the vein") occurs when even a drop of a vesicant chemo agent escapes the tubing, and contacts body tissue. Extravasation is also called a "chemo leak" or a "chemo spill."

Vesicant chemotherapy agents are administered intravenously via a catheter that is inserted into the dog's vein. The drug is delivered via the catheter to ensure that the fluid does not contact the dog's tissue outside of the vein. If the drug contacts tissue or skin of the dog or the veterinarian, there are dire results.

The IV chemo agents that can cause the most dangerous extravasation are the vesicants—the drugs that can result in chemical burns. These include doxorubicin, mitoxantrone, epirubicin, paclitaxel, vinblastine, vincristine, and vinorelbine. The most severe extravasation can result from a doxorubicin (Adriamycin) leak.

Extravasation does not happen often, but it does happen. It can occur even with the most careful medical team, with a staff member staring at the IV site for the entire length of the treatment. An IV tube can back up; a vein can collapse. The damage may not be visible right away, or for as long as ten days. The leaked agent proceeds on a path of destruction that is not easily stopped.

For weeks or months, the agent continues to destroy skin, tendon, and ligament. The tissue turns black, becomes very tough, dies, and drops off. Eventually, the bone is exposed. Often the end result is amputation. My heart goes out to anyone who has to make the heartrending decision to amputate the leg of a dog that is already fighting cancer.

*It is inexcusable that most owners who experience
the nightmare of extravasation have never heard of it.
Any veterinarian giving chemotherapy to a dog
should explain extravasation to the owner.*

One medication has been approved to help resolve extravasations. It is currently not available, but ask your vet about Totect® (dexrazoxane).

Contact with chemo drugs presents a danger to veterinarians and clinic staff as well. Every member of a veterinary team administering intravenous chemotherapy with a vesicant drug wears latex gloves to ensure that the agent does not contact their skin.

Some clinics use a delivery system called PhaSeal® when administering IV chemo drugs, to protect the clinic staff during administration. I have noticed charges for PhaSeal only recently on the invoices. I don't know if the size of the dog has any effect on the price for this tool, but one clinic charged $37.00 for PhaSeal (for a ninety-two pound dog), while another clinic charged $84.15 for PhaSeal (for a fifty-seven pound dog).

▷ **Riley's Story**
A Magic Bullet Fund dog called Riley was in treatment for lymphoma. Riley's owner described a sore near the chemo injection site and e-mailed photos of it to me, and I explained extravasation to her. She had never heard of extravasation or a chemo leak, and was horrified that Riley might lose her leg while beating lymphoma.

I called Riley's oncologist to discuss the possibility of an extravasation. The veterinarian insisted that Riley had not experienced a chemo leak. He said that he would never send a dog home if a chemo leak had occurred.

Nonetheless, Riley's sore progressed during the following two months, looking more and more like an extravasation, until a one-inch length of her leg bone was visible. Sadly, Riley came out of remission and passed away at that point and so there was no further discussion about extravasation.

118

During IV chemotherapy treatments, dogs must not wriggle or move. When a dog is aggressive or very fearful, it can be difficult to administer chemotherapy. For an aggressive or fearful dog, sedation may be necessary during IV chemo treatments to protect the dog from extravasation and to allow the medical team to provide treatment safely.

Sedation can be as simple as giving your dog pills before you leave home. Ask your veterinarian for a sedative, such as diazepam, which you can give your dog twenty minutes before the treatment begins. If your dog is too large for you to carry, sedation should be given at the clinic instead.

For aggressive or fearful dogs, there are pill-form protocols that can be given at home instead of IV chemotherapy. Periodic trips to the clinic, perhaps once a month, will be needed for a quick checkup and blood test.

These protocols provide a somewhat shorter survival time, but in some cases they prove to be just as effective. If your dog is aggressive or fearful, ask your veterinarian to review these treatments with you.

If your dog has no aggression or anxiety issues and will remain still with a vet tech keeping him calm, there should not be any need for sedation or anesthesia. A clinic that routinely sedates or even anesthetizes dogs for chemo treatments may be trying to speed up an assembly line and treat more dogs. Most dogs are fine during treatments with no sedation, and of course sedation should not be given unless necessary.

There is an excellent article about extravasation, including prevention and a very effective medical response. It was written by Alice Villalobos, DVM, for *Veterinary Practice News*. Read this article and provide your veterinarian with a copy of the printout: www.Helpyourdogfightcancer.com/extravasation.shtml.

▷ *Ginger's Story*

A man applied to the Magic Bullet Fund for financial assistance. His dog, Ginger, was having chemotherapy for lymphoma. Ginger's vet called me from the super market. I was straining to hear her between her comments about the produce and her order at the deli counter.

She said she was working for a pharmaceutical company, was no longer a practicing veterinarian, but was doing her friend a favor by giving his dog low-cost chemotherapy treatments.

I asked what clinic she used for the treatments. She said she was treating Ginger in her van, in the parking lot of the company where she and Ginger's dad worked, during their lunch break. I nearly fell off my chair. They all sat in the van with dad holding Ginger's leg still. The veterinarian said she had "a real scare" during a recent treatment because the owner expressed anxiety that Ginger was going to move her leg and he wouldn't be able to hold it still.

I was horrified. I told Ginger's dad that the Magic Bullet Fund would help, but only if he arranged for treatment in an animal hospital or clinic, by a practicing vet. We could not help as long as treatment was being given in this very dangerous (and ridiculous) manner.

Toxicity

Doxorubicin (Adriamycin; Adria) is a powerful drug included in many chemotherapy protocols for lymphoma, hemangiosarcoma, osteosarcoma, and other cancers. Some dogs tolerate Adria with no ill effects at all, and others have severe side effects.

This drug has acquired the nickname "red death." Each chemotherapy agent is given a bright color, so that hopefully no mistakes will be made in selecting the wrong bag of drug to be used. This drug happens to be red. It is called "red death" because it is such a good killer of cancer cells.

Adria is cardiotoxic. After a certain amount has been given, it causes cardiomyopathy and congestive heart failure. There is a prescribed lifetime maximum of doxorubicin that can be given. The rule of thumb is that no more than five treatments can be given at the recommended dose.

If there is a sign that a dog has heart damage at any point during the protocol (even before the first Adria treatment has been given), This drug should be permanently discontinued.

There is evidence that injections of Zinecard® (dexrazoxane) can protect the heart from Adria side effects, given intravenously as infusion just before the Adria drug is administered.

Cytoxan is included in many chemotherapy protocols. It can be given as a pill or intravenously. In either form, it can be damaging to the bladder, although most dogs tolerate it well. Help your dog expel the drug when it has cycled to the bladder. Take him outside to urinate one hour after a cytoxan treatment.

The *platins* (cisplatin and carboplatin) are damaging to the kidneys. Cisplatin is rarely used for dogs because of its very high toxicity. Carboplatin is much less damaging, and much more commonly used, particularly for bone cancers.

Multi-drug Resistance (MDR)

When a dog is diagnosed with cancer, corticosteroids such as prednisone or prednisolone are often prescribed. Putting a dog on a daily dose of corticosteroids may be the first step in starting a chemotherapy protocol.

Putting a dog on a daily dose of corticosteroids may be a palliative measure. If you decline chemotherapy for your dog, the veterinarian will probably recommend daily corticosteroids as a palliative treatment. Prednisone alone does not kill cancer, but it can suppress the cancer for a few months.

> *Prednisone alone causes multi-drug resistance (MDR).*
> *After a dog has been given corticosteroids alone,*
> *combination chemotherapy may not be effective.*

Prednisone is included in most chemotherapy protocols. However, when a dog with lymphoma is given a corticosteroid like prednisone, you must start the chemo treatments quickly thereafter. If chemotherapy does not begin for two weeks, this will lower the chances of chemotherapy being effective.

Multi-drug Resistance Gene Mutation (MDR-1)

Some dogs have the MDR-1 gene mutation. Chemotherapy drugs that are used regularly and safely for other dogs can be very dangerous to them. These are some of the most powerful drugs against cancer. If a cancer cannot be stopped using other drugs, it may be necessary to use these, but carefully.

Every dog has two MDR-1 genes. For a dog with one abnormal (mutant) MDR-1 gene, drugs such as vincristine, vinblastine, and doxorubicin can cause severe side effects. If used, these drugs are administered at only 75 percent of the recommended dosages.

For a dog with two mutant MDR-1 genes, these drugs are toxic and can cause death. If used at all, the dosages should be reduced to 50 percent of the recommended doses.

Breeds that most often carry this genetic mutation, in order of incidence, are collie, long-haired whippet, mini Australian Shepherd, Australian Shepherd, Silken Windhound, McNab, Shetland Sheepdog, English Shepherd, herding breed cross, German Shepherd, Old English Sheepdog, Border Collie, and in dogs mixed with any of these breeds.

You can test for the mutation at home. All you need is a test kit (about $70.00) from Washington State College of Veterinary Medicine, 509-335-3745. Use the kit to submit a cheek swab or a couple of drops of blood and your dog's DNA will be tested for the MDR-1 gene mutation.

Treatment Failure

Certain cancers typically respond to particular treatments, but "typically" does not mean "in every case." If your dog has a type of cancer that typically responds to a certain treatment, and your dog is given that treatment, be optimistic that it will work. While being optimistic, keep in mind that in some percentage of cases, "typically successful" treatments fail.

The cancer may be so advanced or so aggressive that no treatment will stop it without also stopping the life of the patient. The cancer may be resistant to treatment.

Whatever the reason, if the first treatment plan fails, you can try another version of the treatment, or another type of treatment altogether (surgery/chemotherapy/radiation, another approach, or a clinical trial).

When remission is not achieved, chemotherapy dosages may be raised, but doing so raises the risk of toxicity, side effects, and death. Your veterinarian will suggest abandoning the agents in the protocol, since they are not working, and switching to a chemotherapy protocol that uses different agents. Dogs can remain in partial remission for a long time.

It is exceedingly difficult to "give up," but there should be a stopping point, for the benefit of your dog's quality of life. Ultimately, after treatment failure, your veterinarian should recommend palliative care.

If you're not ready to give up the fight, there may still be options to explore. Look into clinical trials. Trials often seek out dogs that have been resistant to standard therapies. The development of a new protocol often begins at a veterinary school where veterinary oncologists select a new combination of agents, a new treatment schedule, and/or a variation of dosages.

Ask a holistic veterinarian about alternative therapies that might help your dog. Explore the library and the Internet for new approaches.

Chemo Costs

There are ways to make a chemotherapy protocol more affordable. Veterinary specialists in chemotherapy routinely make revisions in treatment plans. Revisions can also be made because of financial constraints.

Treatment is often postponed for a week or more, when a dog's white cell count is low. Dosages of the chemotherapy drugs are often reduced, when a dog is sensitive to the drugs and becomes ill after each treatment. I am always surprised when this happens, but for the dogs in the fund, there have been many instances of a treatment being postponed for a week because the veterinarian is on vacation.

The veterinarians are constantly tweaking protocols for academic purposes, to discover a new variation that will work just as well or better as the known protocols.

A protocol *can* be tweaked to make it more affordable. Especially if doing so will make it possible for your dog to have treatment. For example, request that all dosages be reduced to 75 or 80 percent of the recommended dosages. Or request that treatments be scheduled less frequently, such as every ten days or two weeks instead of every week.

There may be fees for antiemetic (anti-nausea) drugs on your invoice. These are great for dogs that experience nausea after chemo treatments, but many dogs do not. If your veterinarian is giving these prophylactically, you can elect to bypass the antiemetic to lower the treatment fee. Then, if you find that your dog vomits or refuses to eat after treatments, you can request that an antiemetic drug be added in.

The biggest fee on the list may be the actual chemo drug. It is not unusual for a clinic to charge the client triple the acquisition cost of the chemo drugs or more.

When a dog in the fund is having chemo, the clinic sends me estimates. When the fees are high, I try to purchase the drugs from a distributor and have them shipped to the clinic. The fund orders and pays for the drugs, and the distributor ships to the clinic. It is just as though the clinic had placed the order, but some clinics refuse to allow me to do this.

Following is a chart showing the fees charged at various clinics across the country, for dogs in the fund to have one chemo treatment with the drug Adriamycin.

Dog's weight (pounds)	Clinic pays for the drug	Clinic charges the owner (for drug only)	Total fee for treatment
14	$13 - 15	46.36	348.74
14	$13 - 15	17.00	316.27
24	$13 - 15	132.00	591.52
38	$32 - 36	249.55	742.55
42	$32 - 36	79.30	421.85
50	$32 - 36	370.00	900.89
60	$32 - 36	48.30	247.80
61	$32 - 36	163.50	381.00
65	$32 - 36	72.00	490.28
68	$32 - 36	340.00	594.00
90	$32 - 36	52.02	485.02
106	$50 - 70	340.00	594.00
117	$50 - 70	387.70	659.53

Some clinics routinely allow owners to order chemo drugs for their dog from a pharmacy or a distributor. If your clinic wants to help you and wants to make it possible for you to afford treatment for your dog, they will allow you to lower the fees by purchasing the drugs yourself.

Although it is possible for a clinic to allow the client to order drugs and give the appearance of being helpful, while continuing to overcharge for the drug. On some treatment estimates, the fee for the drug is lower, but the fees for other tasks, such as "Catheter Placement" or "Chemo Nurse," or "Pha-Seal" are astronomical. When charges are assigned to other items, omitting the fee for the drug will be much less helpful. Then, if the fund (or the owner) purchases the drug and deducts the fee from the invoice, much less is being saved.

> *It is important for veterinarians*
> *not to judge a client's desire to save money*
> *as disloyalty to the practice.*

Find out if your clinic will allow you to purchase the drugs from a pharmacy, and have them delivered to the clinic. If so, call local and mail-order pharmacies to compare prices. You will place the order and the pharmacy will call the clinic to get the prescription from your vet. You will order, pay the pharmacy, and deduct the fee for chemo drug from your invoice. When your dog has treatment, your vet will use the drugs you had shipped rather than the clinic stock.

Drug Prices

I viewed a tutorial offered by one of the many companies that teaches success strategies to veterinary practice managers and staff. One of the lessons concerning "Pricing Strategy" states that the clinic should understand that pet care expense is an increasing percentage of a client's income. Therefore, it is understandable that pet owners will search for better deals.

Further, it says, the online threat of lower drug prices at pharmacies or online pharmacies will not go away. If the clinics ignore it, they will lose income as well as goodwill between client and clinic.

In conclusion, the tutorial suggests that it is better, from a client relationship point of view, for the clinic to take a proactive approach. The tutorial suggests that the clinic sacrifice some drug revenue, in order to retain the client's goodwill. Concentrate on what you are good at and maximize revenue from the services you provide as veterinarians.

The AVMA recently released a series of reports on the veterinary field, including a "2015 AVMA Report on Veterinary Capacity." The summary provided by the AVMA of this report says,

> *"According to the Bureau of Labor Statistics, the fees charged for veterinary services has risen, on average, 5.3 percent annually every year since 1997. The prices people have paid for the same bundle of veterinary services have thus doubled since 1997. In contrast, all other market prices have risen much slower, between 2 percent and 3 percent, on average, during the same period."*

8

Side Effects to Cancer and to Treatment

Most medical treatments have risks and possible side effects. Some are serious or life threatening. Others are minor, easily tolerated or can be remedied quickly if they do occur. When considering cancer treatment for a dog, an owner should be fully informed of all possible outcomes. Discuss treatment options with your vet and ask what is known about the success rate of the treatment. Also ask what the possible side effects are, and how likely your dog is to experience each of them. Ask what will happen if he does have the side effects.

Before we look at the side effects of cancer treatment, I will explain a group of syndromes that are caused by cancer.

Paraneoplastic Syndromes

Paraneoplastic syndromes are side effects not of treatment, but of cancer itself. These syndromes can arise from the cancer, regardless of whether or not treatment has been given.

Sometimes a cancer is discovered and treated successfully only to discover that the dog is suffering from a paraneoplastic syndrome that cannot be controlled.

Sometimes, especially in the cancers that are more difficult to diagnose, cancer is not discovered until after the paraneoplastic syndrome has been diagnosed.

Cachexia and Anorexia

If a dog fighting cancer experiences drastic weight loss, this may be cause for alarm. Your veterinarian will talk to you about cancer cachexia and cancer anorexia.

Cancer cachexia (ka-KEX-ia) is a condition that can develop secondary to cancer, as a neoplastic syndrome. A cachectic dog experiences drastic and progressive weight loss regardless of the quality or quantity of food eaten. He becomes unable to metabolize nutrients, and eventually reaches a state of severe malnutrition.

Once cachexia has developed, it is extremely hard to reverse. A dog may actually have a cure or remission from cancer and die due to cachexia. Some studies indicate that a low-carbohydrate, high-fat diet may protect a dog from cachexia. High levels of omega-3 fatty acids in the diet may decrease the chances that a dog with cancer will develop cancer cachexia.

Cancer anorexia can also develop secondary to cancer. Cancer anorexia can be reversed more easily than cancer cachexia. It's similar to cachexia in that the dog undergoes extreme weight loss, but in this case the weight loss is due to the dog's refusal to eat.

If a dog is eating and losing weight, the cause may be cachexia. If a dog is not eating and losing weight, the case may be anorexia.

Hypercalcemia

Hypercalcemia means there is a higher than normal concentration of calcium in the blood. Hypercalcemia develops as a paraneoplastic complication of late-stage cancer, most commonly in T-cell LSA, apocrine gland anal sac adenocarcinoma, breast cancer, and multiple myeloma but in other cancers as well.

Hypercalcemia can be diagnosed by a blood test. When hypercalcemia is discovered and treated early, it can be reversed.

If not treated early, hypercalcemia can lead to kidney dysfunction. The end result is usually coma and/or renal failure.

If your dog is hypercalcemic, be sure that no supplements you are giving him contain Vitamin D. Ask your vet about giving your dog IV fluids and a concurrent low dose of Lasix® (furosemide). This may be helpful, but unless the underlying cause is addressed, any benefit will be short lived.

CNS Paraneoplastic Syndromes

Cancer cells can invade the central nervous system (CNS). This is seen in cancers that are neurologically based, such as a brain tumor, or from metastasized cancer cells from a tumor elsewhere. Some cancers create lesions in the peripheral nerves, causing weakness, lameness, or paralysis.

CNS paraneoplastic syndromes may be reversible with early intervention, but become irreversible over time.

Surgery Side Effects

Surgery that requires anesthesia always carries a risk. When surgery is needed for a dog with cardiac or respiratory issues, additional monitoring can be set up to alert the surgeon if the dog is in distress. Other specialists may be present or on call for consultation during the surgical procedure.

Infection is another possible outcome resulting from surgery. Follow your vet's instructions to keep the incision site clean. Call your vet right away if the skin near the wound becomes very swollen or changes color. Call your vet if the wound emits an odor or if fluids such as pus or blood are leaking from it.

Post-operative pain medications are usually dispensed after a surgery, for the owner to provide at home. There are possible side effects from these medications. Alert your vet if your dog cannot be awakened after you give pain medication. Alert your vet of blood in the stool or vomiting, or any unusual swelling.

Just as people react differently to pain medications, so do dogs. You may need to increase or decrease the dosage according to your dog's reaction. He should not be crying from pain and he should not be in a coma. Ask your vet what the upper and lower limits are that would be appropriate to give your dog, and then you can adjust the dosage at home according to his response.

Radiation Therapy Side Effects

The most common side effect of radiation therapy may be skin burns. The burns can be severe, and healing can be difficult or impossible. The higher the dose and more aggressive the treatment schedule, the higher the risk of burns and the more severe the burns tend to be.

This side effect is difficult to control because the burns often don't appear until after all of the treatments have been completed. Once burns do appear, they may worsen before improving and carry a possibility of infection. Radiation burns should be treated by a veterinarian.

Radiation therapy may be ruled out for a cancer in the head because of the damage it can do to the brain. When applied to the head, there are two common side effects. These are faucitis mucositis (an inflammation of the tissue lining the mouth) and dry eye (irritation of tissue around the eyes, with decreased tear production).

Radiation therapy may cause severe bladder irritation or "radiation cystitis," which requires prompt treatment by a veterinarian, as well as the development of blood clots. Like most cancer treatment, radiation therapy can cause myelosuppression.

Chemo (Drug-Specific) Side Effects

Each chemotherapy drug has side effects that were experienced by a percentage of the test group while the drug was going through trials for FDA approval. Some are common, and others occur in only a small percentage of patients. These are only statistics. Some dogs are sensitive to all of the agents and become ill from each treatment. Others suffer side effects only to particular agents. Others seem immune to side effects from any agent and can tolerate every treatment without any sign of illness.

Some of the chemotherapy drugs have unique, serious side effects. They do not occur in most dogs, but they are well known and documented. Owners should be aware of these possibilities. With this knowledge, when an adverse reaction occurs, the remedies can be given and adjustments can be made to a chemo protocol quickly.

Prednisone

Most protocols include prednisone (or prednisolone) given every day at first and then every other day. It is generally phased out after a few weeks. This drug can cause excessive drinking, urination, and panting. Prednisone can be hard on the lining of the stomach. Break the tablet into pieces so that the whole pill doesn't sit on your dog's stomach wall. If the side effects are unmanageable, talk to your vet about reducing the dosage.

Bullet reacted badly to prednisone. With Dr. Porzio's agreement, I lowered the dose to 75 percent and then to half, but he was still having severe diarrhea, enormous thirst, and accidents in the house. After three weeks, I stopped giving him prednisone entirely because Dr. Porzio said that lowering it any more would mean giving him an amount that was below the therapeutic level. Bullet was given no prednisone for the rest of his protocol, even though it is included in most protocols for canine lymphoma.

During the first phase of a chemo protocol, a dog may be given prednisone as well as cytoxan. When administering cytoxan, many veterinary oncologists also give furosemide to protect the kidneys. Prednisone plus furosemide can result in a tremendous amount of urination.

▷ **Franke Swinarski's Story**

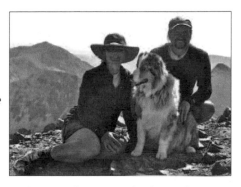

Cindy and Ken Swinarski's dog Franke was a 4-year-old Aussie with lymphoma. Cindy had questions about Franke's treatment plan, so she found me at www.AskLaurie.us and scheduled a phone call. We talked about Franke's medical treatment and home care.

Later, Cindy emailed to tell me that Franke, given both prednisone and cytoxan, had to be taken outside to pee very often. Nothing new about that, it is a very common problem for dogs in cancer treatment. But Cindy thought up what I consider a brilliant method of managing this problem, so I am sharing it here.

Cindy emailed, "I tried sleeping on the deck and about froze to death. Now I just drink a ton of water before I go to bed and all during the night, so that when I have to wake up to go to the bathroom I let him out. That's working!

Thanks again for your sincere support, help and advice. It keeps me from having panic attacks."

Cindy Swinarski, Scottsdale, Arizona

Vincristine (Oncovin®) Neuropathy

Certain chemo agents cause peripheral neurotoxicity. This occurs when nerve coatings are stripped away from the nerves. Chemotherapy agents such as vincristine, carboplatin, cisplatin, and paclitaxel are known to cause peripheral neurotoxicity and peripheral neuropathy.

Chemotherapy-induced peripheral neuropathy (CIPN) is the loss of feeling in a limb. Dogs cannot tell us, "I am feeling pins and needles in my rear left leg." Therefore, CIPN is usually not diagnosed in dogs until it has progressed to cause lameness or limping.

Is the loss of feeling accompanied by pain? Because dogs aren't able to describe sensations, I looked for a description of the effects on humans. People report that CIPN is painful. In human cancer treatment, therapy with the offending drug is generally discontinued when a patient develops CIPN.

The following was provided by Charles L. Loprinzi, MD, professor of oncology at the Mayo Clinic College of Medicine, Rochester, Minnesota.

> *"Pain in the hands and feet, muscle cramps, numbness and tingling in the fingertips and toes have been reported in over 50 percent of patients receiving vincristine therapy; affected patients may have changes in their ability to feel things, to detect sharpness, and to sense temperature ... Recovery from the neuropathy may take up to two years, may worsen after vincristine is stopped, and it is not always reversible."*

CIPN may be reversible when treatment with the drug causing it is stopped as soon as it is discovered. If your dog is having treatment with vincristine or the other chemo drugs causing this side effect, do not ignore the early signs. Watch for limping or knuckling. Watch for difficulty standing up or walking. If your dog starts to limp or has difficulty moving one or both rear legs, alert your veterinarian immediately, and discuss with him the possibility that it might be CIPN.

Glutathione and vitamin E may be given prophylactically in an attempt to avoid this side effect while a neurotoxic drug is given.

This side effect is dose related. The higher the dose, the more likely the side effect. Once this occurs, the drug causing it should be stopped. If not stopped entirely, dosages should be reduced by 25 or 50 percent.

Cytoxan (cyclophosphamide)

This chemotherapy drug is included in many protocols, in pill or intravenous form. The drug is much less expensive in pill form, and it can be given at home by the owner without a visit to the clinic.

Cytoxan causes bladder side effects, most notably hemorrhagic cystitis with bloody urine. When given cytoxan, dogs are also treated with furosemide to flush the urinary system and protect the bladder. It may help to have your dog urinate one hour after treatment with this drug.

Adriamycin (doxorubicin)

This chemotherapy agent is cardiotoxic and can cause cardiomyopathy quickly or months after treatment. A maximum lifetime dose of five treatments is generally accepted as safe, but some dogs can tolerate more and others are not able to tolerate this amount. The supplement L-carnitine may help to protect the heart from this drug.

Your vet can administer dexrazoxane (Zinecard®) before each Adria treatment. This may protect the heart, but it has its own side effects, most of which are allergy related. Other negatives of giving a dog Zinecard are that it may add to the myelosuppression that Adriamycin causes, and it is a very expensive drug.

Chemo Side Effects

Every dog is different. Your dog may not have the typical reactions to chemotherapy treatments. He may have reactions that are not included in the list of common side effects.

When serious side effects occur, manage them right away. Inform your veterinarian or oncologist immediately. He might prescribe medication, or there might be something you can do at home to resolve the reaction. He might say to bring your pet into the clinic right away, or he might say not to worry because the reaction is normal and self-limiting.

You have a "team" of experts contributing to your dog's well-being. Call them for help with side effects. In time, you'll learn who is most accessible with the best solutions. Make a note in your journal about the episode, including what it was that finally helped and who suggested it.

Make a note in your journal so you will know what to do the next time this reaction occurs.

Sidestep future side effects by adjusting the protocol. History repeats itself. You can expect your dog to have the same reaction the next time he receives this drug. Ask your dog's veterinarian to "discount" the dosage to of that drug to 75 or 80 percent of the recommended dose for all subsequent treatments. Often a dog will tolerate the drug at a lower dose. If your dog still has severe side effects to a lower dose, talk to the veterinarian about excluding this agent from the protocol and replacing it with a different chemo agent.

Vomiting and Nausea

Antiemetics can prevent vomiting in dogs undergoing chemotherapy. If your dog vomits after treatment, tell your veterinarian. Before your dog's next treatment, he can be pretreated with an antiemetic (see below).

Excessive vomiting can cause dehydration. To test for dehydration, pick up the skin on the scruff of your dog's neck, where a pup's mother would grab on to carry her pup. Then let go. If the skin doesn't fall down flat on your dog's neck within a two to three seconds, he may be dehydrated. Call your veterinarian.

Also call if there is any blood in the vomitus, if vomiting persists for more than two days, or if your dog vomits more than three times in a twenty-four-hour period.

The vomitus may contain traces of the toxic chemicals that were not fully absorbed into your dog's system. Clean up as best you can wearing protective gloves. Then, dissipate the vomitus by pouring water over it so that other animals don't eat it.

- ▶ Prescription (Rx): Antiemetic such as Cerenia® (maropitant citrate), Reglan®, Zofran®, or Anzemet®. Some dogs have allergic reactions to these drugs.
- ▶ Over-the-counter (OTC): Pepto-Bismol®, particularly after chemo with Adriamycin is given. Check with your vet first.
- ▶ Pepcid® AC (check with your veterinarian first.)
- ▶ Other: Ginger is a natural remedy for nausea. Pumpkin may help when your pup is nauseous. Canned mashed pumpkin can be found in any supermarket.

▸ L-Glutamine: If your dog takes this regularly, you can double the amount while vomiting persists.

▸ Nux Vomica 6C

Diarrhea

Again, clean up! Most chemotherapy agents are expelled from the dog's body through urine or feces. Some are still "active" after being expelled. Clean up after your dog so that other dogs, cats, or people do not make contact with an expelled chemo agent that may still be active. Wear latex gloves—active agent can be absorbed through the skin.

Watch for mucous in the stool, which can indicate infection. You will see a loose stool that glistens or hangs before falling to the ground, or a shiny liquid stool. If you suspect there is mucous in your dog's stool, tell your veterinarian.

Projectile diarrhea. This is a shocking experience for the owner, from personal experience. Try to stay out of the spray zone—otherwise, treat the same as ordinary diarrhea.

▸ Prescription (Rx): Flagyl® (metronidozole)

▸ OTC: Pepto-Bismol; Imodium®; Lomotil. Check with your veterinarian before giving these remedies.

▸ Other: Give your dog L-Glutamine! This is an essential amino acid with no negative effects even in high doses. It is the best way to avoid or minimize damage to the intestines from chemo, which is what causes diarrhea after treatment.

▸ Acidophilus and bifidus: As chewable tablets or in organic yogurt.

▸ Temporarily decrease oil (fatty acids) as supplements or in food.

▸ Add potato, brown rice, sweet potato, or pumpkin to the diet, until the diarrhea stops. Also sprinkle a high-fiber bran cereal onto your dog's food.

▸ Pectin: Mix a teaspoon of powdered pectin with filtered water in a needle-less syringe and empty it slowly into your dog's mouth.

▸ Do not give vitamin C or CoQ10.

Bloody Diarrhea

The lining of a dog's intestines can be damaged by chemotherapy agents. If you see any blood in your dog's stool, notify your veterinarian.

Dark-red or black-looking stools may be caused by dried blood, which occurs if the bleeding is high in the GI tract (in the stomach). This can indicate an ulcer. Red-colored stools contain liquid blood, usually from the lower GI tract (small or large intestines).

▸ Bovine colostrum

▸ Same as list for diarrhea

Inappetence (Not Eating)

It is common for dogs with cancer, especially those having chemotherapy, to go through changes in appetite. This can be very challenging for the cook! If your dog turns his nose up at his dinner or does not eat anything for an entire day, do not panic. This is why one of my mottos is "Keep him fat." However, if he refuses to eat for more than a day or two, then you need to take action.

Another possible explanation for loss of appetite is the presence of an infection. Check your dog's temperature. Normal is 100 to 102.5 degrees, so alert your veterinarian if your dog's temperature is above 103 degrees Fahrenheit. If there is no elevated fever, then most likely he is not eating because of the cancer and the treatments. Work on getting your dog to eat.

Start with foods that are healthy and cancer-conscious, but resort to anything. The longer he doesn't eat, the less inclined he will be to start eating—in other words, "not eating" can become habitual.

Try canned herring, cat food, baby food, or liverwurst. Offer him a smorgasbord and hope that he will like one of your offerings. Put small portions of several different meals out to see which one he will eat. Feed that to him, whatever it is, as long as he keeps eating it. For about a month, Bullet would eat nothing other than beef liver.

Feed frozen. Heating food to combat nausea is often recommended. If it works, great! In my experience this is not effective. I do know that when I am nauseous the smell of food makes me more nauseous. I have had much more success getting dogs to eat by feeing frozen food, so that it does not have any odor at all.

▸ Prescription (Rx): antiemetics may be prescribed since loss of appetite may be due to nausea.

▸ OTC: Pepcid® AC, Rescue Remedy

▸ Other: Bullet's "Frozen Fishies," cottage cheese, ginger, garlic

Bullet had stopped eating. I tried anything and everything, but he had no interest whatsoever in food. During one spell of inappetence, he'd lost fifteen pounds, dropping from eight-five pounds to seventy. I have no doubt that Bully's Frozen Food Diet saved his life (see "Feeding Frozen").

I discovered another method to get Bullet to eat. I can't explain how I happened to discover it. I placed the food bowl within Bullet's reach, and I inserted a finger into his ear (sometimes one in each ear) and rubbed gently, back and forth. Somewhere within the nooks and crannies, I found a particular spot that seemed to prompt a reflexive eating response! If your dog stops eating, try this. Perhaps it will work for your dog, too.

After Bullet's first dramatic weight loss, I made a decision to "keep him fat." I tried to maintain him at about five pounds over his perfect weight. If he was carrying a few extra pounds, I would not panic about a one- or two-day fast.

"Flat Out"

When a dog is non-responsive, not eating, and hardly moving, I call this condition "flat out." Dr. Ruslander advises that it's urgent to notify your veterinarian if this condition appears because it could indicate neutropenia (a very low WBC and neutrophil count) or sepsis (high levels of toxins in the blood).

If a dog is febrile (has a temperature above 103 degrees Fahrenheit), this is a life-threatening emergency. Dr. Cotter says that when a dog is febrile, bactericidal antibiotics, such as a combination of gentamicin and cephalothin, or fluoroquinolones, are given intravenously until the neutrophil count rises. In most cases, the dog will recover within two to three days.

- ▸ Your veterinarian will check your dog's white blood cell count and neutrophil count
- ▸ Check your dog's temperature
- ▸ Get him to eat! Try anything and everything. Appetite enhancers are not especially effective in dogs. Try Bullet's Frozen Fishies, see chapter called "What's Your Dog Eating?"
- ▸ Rescue Remedy, Vitamin B-12

Bullet's chemotherapy began with two treatments of doxorubicin. He showed no reaction at all to the first, except that he threw up lots of clear fluid a day later. After the second he became extremely ill. Bullet was flat out 24/7, sometimes crying quietly. He needed my help to go outside to pee. There was blood in his stool, and he was vomiting. I thought it would be a miracle if he pulled through. He did not have a fever, his white blood cell count (WBC) was low but not dangerously low, and he was not dehydrated. I could have decided to end the fight, but I felt that he had it in him to recover. I simply waited it out and did what I could to help him recover from the chemo side effects.

One day, a friend said, "Many people whose pets have cancer would request euthanasia for their dog rather than put him through chemotherapy." Indeed I did question my decision to keep going, then and many other times. Each time Bullet became ill with side effects, I decided "not yet." I had no way of knowing whether Bullet would survive the episode. If he had not, would my decision have been the wrong one? In the absence of a crystal ball, I had to trust my intuition.

Caring for a dog through cancer treatment can be like a roller coaster ride. Bullet and I weathered many setbacks. Each time, I knew that he might not recover. I watched him very carefully for any sign that he was in distress or that he would not recover. And I continued to do whatever I could to help him recover.

Difficulty Breathing

Some dogs have allergic reactions to certain chemotherapy agents in the form of respiratory distress. This may manifest as rasping, wheezing, or reverse sneezing. Notify your oncologist or your veterinarian right away—anaphylactic shock is possible and can be fatal. If the cause is a sensitivity to a particular chemotherapy agent, the dosage of the agent may be decreased. If the symptoms are caused by an allergic reaction, use of the agent is discontinued entirely.

Prescription (Rx): Clavamox®, an antibiotic. Dr. Cotter says that antibiotics will help resolve this condition if it's caused by a respiratory infection such as pneumonia.

Swelling

This may signal an allergic reaction to a chemotherapy agent or to the long-term use of prednisone. Swelling may also be caused by edema due to a tumor, or by heart failure.

Inform your veterinarian immediately if you notice swelling.

Anemia

Although anemia (insufficient red blood cell count) is not a typical chemotherapy side effect, many dogs in cancer treatment become mildly anemic as a reaction to the immunosuppressive nature of chemotherapy. However, if the cancer has infiltrated the bone marrow and is not in remission, the red cells, white cells, and platelets all become insufficient. When this occurs, the prognosis is poor.

> ▶ Prescription (Rx): Procrit® is often prescribed. Aranesp® (darbepo-etin alfa) treats anemia caused by chemotherapy
> ▶ OTC: Chlorophyll drops (with mint, if your dog has bad breath!)

Hair Loss

Fur clipped or shaved during chemotherapy will grow back, but more slowly than normal. If you want to keep your dog's coat looking beautiful, ask your vet not to shave any more of your dog's coat than is necessary. This is particularly important for a dog with a big furry coat, when the patches will be very obvious.

While most dogs don't typically lose their hair to chemo, it is common for dogs to lose their whiskers early on and to experience some hair loss when chemotherapy continues for more than a few months.

> ▶ Brush well to remove loose and dead hair or fur.
> ▶ Nettles (dry herb flakes, crumbled on food) and Silica 500 (found in health food stores) may help your dog regrow his coat.

Bullet lost all of his whiskers at month three of his chemotherapy protocol, but the rest of his coat remained intact until month seventeen. At that time, with only one month of chemotherapy left, his undercoat fell out suddenly, in handfuls. For the first time in his life, Bullet was showing pink skin on his belly.

I added supplements to his regimen thought to promote hair

*growth, and the undercoat grew back nicely. Then, just as his under-
coat was growing in again, his guard hair coat dropped out. Bullet's
head and neck retained the double coat typical of a Northern breed
dog, but the rest of his body was furred only with a soft, downy undercoat. The next time we saw him, Dr. Porzio exclaimed, "The Bullet
looks like a giant chinchilla!"*

*For the rest of his life, Bullet had no guard hair coat except around
his neck. His body was soft as cotton, and I added the nickname,
"Bunny Boy" to his list of nicknames. I missed watching my fingers
disappear into his deep, luxurious fur, but all in all, this was a very
small price to pay for four and a half years on borrowed time!*

Don't Panic!

Most dogs in chemotherapy do need to miss at least one treatment due
to a low WBC count. Don't worry if a chemotherapy treatment is postponed for a week. One oncologist told me that she and her colleagues have
a theory: When a dog has minor, manageable side effects, it is a sign of
treatment success. It proves that if the chemo drugs are killing off some
healthy cells, they are probably killing lots of cancer cells.

Treat the symptoms and make your dog as comfortable as possible.
Usually the WBC count will recover within a week and the protocol can
continue. If side effects are not severe and can be managed, or if your dog
recovers quickly, treatment will continue according to the plan.

If your dog is acting as though he doesn't feel well, you may decide to
postpone a treatment even if the vet doesn't find any clinical reason to
postpone. Vets make decisions based on a blood test, but you can make it
based on your knowledge of your dog and your observation of him at
home. Pay attention to your intuition, based on your intimate knowledge
of your dog. A sick dog should not be given chemotherapy.

If the white count has fallen low enough to indicate neutropenia, your
dog will require medical treatment at the clinic. He will receive IV fluids
and antibiotics, and will be monitored closely. The drug that caused
neutropenia should not be given again.

If your dog has severe side effects more than once, or if the side effects are so severe that hospitalization is necessary, talk to your vet about revising the protocol. The objective is for chemotherapy to kill the cancer, not the dog. Dr. Porzio said to me many times during Bullet's treatment, "Chemotherapy is not an exact science." Protocols are often customized.

Chemotherapy Revisions

Treatment plans, medications, and schedules can be revised as needed, to give your dog the best chance of beating cancer without suffering severe side effects. If the treatment is not working, or if your dog has severe side effects to the treatment (whether the treatment is working or not), a revision is needed.

You can continue treatment in hopes (against the odds) that your dog will better tolerate subsequent treatments. However, the side effects will most likely continue and worsen unless a change is made.

First, make sure that your veterinarian is pre-medicating your dog with benadryl, for example, before intravenous chemotherapy treatments. Make sure that your vet is giving the drug Adriamycin as an infusion over at least twenty minutes (five to ten minutes for a small dog).

Ask your veterinarian to suggest revisions or another treatment option. If your dog has side effects from one drug in particular, you can give your dog a smaller dose of the offending agent when it appears in the schedule. Discounting the dose of a drug by 20 to 25 percent is common. You may decide to omit that drug entirely and replace it with a different drug when it appears in the protocol. You may decide to schedule treatments every two weeks instead of every week, or every three weeks instead of every two weeks. Or there may be another treatment protocol that's equally effective and that your dog can better tolerate.

If more than one drug is causing severe side effects, you can abandon the protocol and replace it with an entirely different one. The new protocol should not include the chemo drugs that made your dog sick.

Or, you can stop treatment and provide palliative care. Some dogs are simply not be able to tolerate treatment.

Bullet became very ill after treatment with Adriamycin. We tried giving a lower dose at the next treatment, but he again had severe side effects. I chose to exclude Adriamycin from Bullet's protocol after the second dose, even though it was long before his lifetime maximum quantity was reached. From that point on, whenever Adria came up in the protocol, it was substituted by a different chemo agent in the protocol (vincristine or Cytoxan).

Make use of supplements to support medical treatment and improve its potential for success. All dogs in chemotherapy should be given L-Glutamine, an essential amino acid that protects the small intestines from chemo damage. There are no negative effects or adverse reactions to L-Glutamine even at high doses. It will help you avoid the common gastrointestinal side effects of diarrhea and bloody diarrhea.

Anti-inflammatory supplements such as SAMe or Wobenzym® N or Wobenzym® may minimize inflammation. Inflammation is a factor because the uncontrolled cell division that defines cancer is a type of inflammation in itself, and also causes inflammation.

Milk thistle can protect your dog's liver, but be careful using this while also using SAMe. You may think you are helping your dog's liver when you are really over-activating it. Speak to your vet before giving your dog milk thistle.

9

New and Alternative Treatments

Shortly after Bullet's diagnosis, a holistic veterinarian recommended an alternative cancer treatment I had not heard about. I read the literature and asked Dr. Hoskins and Dr. Porzio to read it as well. After hearing their thoughts, I decided against this therapy, even though it just might, some day, turn out to be the "Magic Bullet" against canine lymphoma.

Many alternative therapies for canine cancer are in development or in FDA testing but are not yet approved. Others are treatments that have been available for a long time but are not considered mainstream cancer treatment, nor are they seeking FDA approval.

Choose alternative therapies based on research, test results, empirical data, advice from your team members, and other people who have dogs with cancer. Manufacturers and distributors—those who will gain financially from sales—show testimonials and anecdotal success stories. Look instead for articles about controlled studies showing the success rate of the treatment in peer-reviewed veterinary journals before signing up.

There are always many new treatments for cancer at various stages of development. Some are being studied in petri dishes in laboratories; others are farther along in the process and are being used to treat cancer dogs and/or humans in clinical trials. All of the new therapies have the potential to become effective in the fight against cancer, but few do come to fruition. Many have shown some success in some cases, but have not yet been tested for safety and consistency or fine-tuned for the correct dosages and number of treatments needed for the highest efficacy, lowest toxicity, and fewest side effects.

Trials help to establish all of this and then work out the details of precisely how a tool can be discovered. The farther along the therapy is in the development process, the more realistically you can hope that it might be effective for your dog.

Clinical trials for cancer treatment used on dogs may lead to the development of the treatment for humans. When you choose a treatment in early development for your dog, you are enlisting your dog as a test subject. If you are required to pay for treatment, you may be supporting research, offsetting the costs of research and development in laboratories and pharmaceutical companies, and subsidizing the salaries of doctors, veterinarians, researchers, and others.

Gaining FDA approval and moving a treatment or drug through the arduous approval process costs millions of dollars. There is a small chance that your contributions may lead to a groundbreaking discovery and may benefit your dog. More likely, your contributions will fund cancer research that has a miniscule chance of leading to a breakthrough. The willingness of dog owners to try "anything" to help their dogs survive cancer has created a heyday for companies that develop cancer treatments and drugs, as well as for clinics and veterinarians.

New cutting-edge cancer treatments are often tested on pet dogs before approval. Some of this research is financed by loving owners like you who are only trying to save your dog's life. For example, testing on dogs helped scientists figure out how to reduce the risk of immune system rejection and led to the first successful human bone marrow transplants.

Comparative Oncology

Comparative oncology is the study of cancer across species. For example, veterinary oncologists and human oncologists work together to study and compare the behavior of cancer in dogs versus the behavior of cancer in humans.

This includes comparing responses to cancer treatments in development. Through comparative oncology, it is hoped that more effective cancer treatments will emerge. The objective of comparative oncology is to test new treatments on dogs in order to improve cancer treatment for humans.

The University of California Comprehensive Cancer Center website offers this definition: "In comparative oncology programs, veterinarians collaborate with physicians who treat humans and conduct research using pet dogs and cats. The idea is that what is learned from pets will be applied to human cancer."

In 2006 Sutent® (sunitinib malate) became the first drug ever simultaneously approved by the FDA for use in two different types of human cancer. In 2009, Palladia became the first drug ever approved specifically for treating dogs with cancer. Its success, according to Dr. Cheryl London, DVM and cancer researcher at Ohio State University's Veterinary Medical Center, is due in part because researchers were able to treat dogs first, which greatly helped to inform the design of human studies.

Dogs and people get the same types of cancer, with few exceptions. Treatment provided to dogs with cancer is the same or only marginally different from treatment provided to people with cancer. There is one important difference. The age-old theory comparing "dog years" to "human years" is that a dog's age times seven would be the equivalent human age. This estimated seven-to-one ratio emerged because of an estimate that the average dog lives approximately one seventh as long as the average human lives.

A dog's response to cancer treatment also occurs faster than a human's. This is of great importance and of great use to researchers, treatment specialists, and pharmaceutical companies. The development of new cancer treatments for humans may be expedited tremendously through comparative oncology. A treatment that is not approved for testing on humans may be approved for testing on dogs.

For example, in 2007, a team of researchers in Germany published a study showing some success with mice using the antibiotic tuarolidine (TRD) against melanoma. As a result, TRD is being tested against human osteosarcoma, but it is being tested only on human cell lines, not on actual humans, because the research and development is not far enough along for the FDA to allow its use on humans.

Although it cannot be tested on humans, TRD is being tested on dogs in clinical trials at the University of Oregon. Preliminary clinical trials are testing taurolidine alone and in combination with these two drugs for dogs with osteosarcoma. At this time, TRD is available in the United States only for research purposes.

By studying the effects of a cancer treatment in dogs, researchers can evaluate the potential success of a new drug for humans in an accelerated model (the dog). They can determine the potential success of that treatment in months rather than years.

Some veterinary specialty clinics and veterinary schools are at the forefront of cancer research. They find treatments and drugs in development that they can offer clients who have dogs with cancer. They can offer them because while treatments and drugs used by oncologists who treat humans with cancer are strictly monitored and regulated, while there are very few restrictions on the use of treatments and drugs for veterinary use.

Watch for an upcoming book about comparative oncology by Arlene Weintraub titled *Heal: The Vital Role of Dogs in the Search for Cancer Cures* (ECW Press). Weintraub introduces readers to comparative oncology, focusing on cutting-edge research to find new therapies for cancers similar in dogs and people.

Weintraub's book explores the fascinating and vital role that dogs are playing in the search for a cure for cancer. The author brings the dogs and their human companions to life, to show how man's best friend might be the key to unlocking the mysteries of cancer.

Immunotherapy

Perhaps the most fascinating studies are those that explore the viability of fighting and/or curing cancer through immunotherapy. This is a very complex and fascinating technology that is showing promising signs of success. One treatment in this category is monoclonal antibody therapy.

Monoclonal antibody (mAb) therapy has made substantial contributions to the fight against cancer in recent years. In a process called XenoMouse technology, mice are stimulated to produce large amounts of antibodies. Not just any antibodies, but the specific antibodies that are produced to fight a specific cancer cell in a specific species.

Monoclonal antibodies are therefore disease-specific and species-specific. This means that the mAb for one type of canine cancer is different from the mAb for another type of canine cancer, (disease-specific) and the mAb for a certain cancer in canines is different from the mAb for that same cancer in humans (species-specific).

Once produced, the antibodies are extracted from the mouse and delivered to the cancer patient intravenously. MAbs are "targeted therapies," because they affect very specific cancer cells and do not harm healthy cells. Traditional chemotherapy is not targeted, because it acts on all cells in a certain stage of cell division, including healthy cells.

Three mAbs—Rituxan®, Zevalin®, and Bexxar®—have been approved for use in fighting non-Hodgkin's lymphoma in humans. Herceptin® (trastuzumab) is a mAb that combats breast cancer in humans. These are available and in common use today.

Some medical advances have been accomplished by first testing them on pet dogs. Many new treatments in the theoretical stage are given to dogs to establish response rates, and to find optimal dosage and scheduling for treatments. This important stage of development leading to human cancer treatment has been accomplished using dogs, only to become unavailable to help dogs fight cancer once approved for human use.

The monoclonal antibody developed to fight canine lymphoma was called mAb 231. MAb 231 was available shortly before Bullet's diagnosis. It was used along with chemotherapy, not instead. I was interested to learn more about mAb-231 and searched for information about it. I contacted the laboratory that developed it and the distributor, but people I spoke to said that it had vanished, possibly due to a lack of demand.

An attempt to revive mAb231 was made in 2012, by Dr. Joe Impellizeri DVM, DACVIM, MRCVS, Diplomate- American College of Veterinary Internal Medicine (Oncology), Member, Royal College of Veterinary Surgeons, Veterinary Oncology Services, PLLC, Visiting Scholar-Vassar College, NY and Director, Barrymore Center for Advanced Cancer Therapeutics. I asked Dr. Impellizeri how that project was going, and he said, "We ran into some significant limitations moving forward on 231. I am doubtful it will ever be able to be revived." (email 4/19/2014)

Vaccine Therapies

When Dr. Phil Bergman was adjunct associate faculty member at Memorial Sloan Kettering Cancer Center in New York City, he worked in cooperation with the medical oncologists at Sloan Kettering, including Dr. Jedd D. Wolchock, MD, PhD. In a PBS report titled "Dogs Shed New Light on Cancer Genes in Humans," (March 15, 2007), Dr. Wolchock says about his work with Dr. Bergman, "I saw the opportunity to possibly, in my wildest dreams, help his dogs, but also get some early evidence for safety and efficacy of our vaccine."

The result of this particular collaborative effort was ONCEPT®. This early collaborative effort in the field of comparative oncology resulted in the DNA vaccine for canine melanoma, now available from Merial as ONCEPT® for dogs with melanoma. In 2011, Dr. Bergman received the inaugural "Innovation in Veterinary Medicine" award from Morris Animal Foundation for his work on the melanoma vaccine.

▷ *Kirby Donovan's Story*

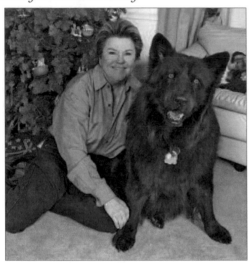

Magic Bullet Fund dog Kirby came to the fund with oral melanoma. Kirby's owner, Blake, researched canine melanoma and found information about a vaccine in development for the treatment of canine melanoma. It was the same DNA vaccine that Dr. Bergman worked on, discussed earlier. Blake brought the information to Dr. Alice Villalobos at the VCA in Hermosa Beach, CA, and she made arrangements to give Kirby treatment with Merial's DNA vaccine, available then only under conditional licensing from the FDA.

Kirby started treatment in July 2007 and did not develop any new CMM tumors. Eight months after treatment began, an x-ray revealed nodules in her lungs. Dr. Bergman said that in addition to fighting CMM, the vaccine may actually slow the progression of secondary lung cancer (cancer metastasized to the lungs). Kirby continued to have DNA vaccine treatments until March 2008, when she passed.
- Blake Donovan, West Hills, California

This highly aggressive cancer spreads very quickly and is resistant to standard therapies. This is a cancer that was considered terminal in the short term, and there was no effective treatment. Dr. Bergman says:

> *"Novel therapies are desperately needed for this extremely malignant tumor. Historically, the median survival time for dogs with advanced CMM given standard treatments was three to six months. However, the median survival time for the dogs treated with surgery or radiation followed by the DNA vaccine is approaching two years."*

Tyrosine Kinase Inhibitors; TKIs

Palladia® (toceranib), Kinavet-CA1® (masitinib), and Gleevec® (imatinib) have been successfully used in dogs. Palladia was celebrated as the first cancer drug approved by the FDA specifically for dogs. All other cancer drugs used for dogs are actually drugs approved for use in human cancer. To date, Palladia has not been used for humans with cancer.

Masitinib has proven efficacy against mast cell cancer in dogs. Studies are underway to find out if it is effective against other types of cancer.

CD40-Activated B-Cell Cancer Vaccine

Researchers at the University of Pennsylvania's School of Veterinary Medicine and School of Medicine have conducted a clinical trial evaluating the safety and efficacy of a cell-based lymphoma vaccine in prolonging overall survival in dogs with lymphoma. One of the researchers, Dr. Nicola Mason, BVetMed, PhD (immunology) DACVIM (internal medicine), explained to me (email, 4/21/14):

> *"The CD40-B cell vaccine is a cell-based vaccine. It consists of the patient's own white blood cells, known as B cells. They are activated outside of the body and loaded with genetic material from the patient's own tumor. These cells are then injected back into the patient where they present tumor antigens to the immune system and stimulate an anti-tumor immune response."*

Dogs with newly diagnosed lymphoma received standard chemotherapy, but not the entire protocol. The treatments continued only until the dog achieved full clinical remission. Then, chemotherapy stopped and the vaccine was given once every three weeks for three treatments. In early results, the vaccinated dogs relapsed with lymphoma at the same time as dogs that did not receive the vaccine.

However, the dogs that had received the vaccine had a much longer second remission following rescue chemotherapy compared to a control group that was treated in the same way but did not receive the vaccination. In the study group of nineteen dogs, fifteen dogs relapsed. Of these, 40 percent of the vaccinated dogs had long-term survival after receiving a standard rescue chemotherapy protocol. Only 7 percent of the control dogs that were not vaccinated and received the same standard rescue chemotherapy protocol had long-term survival.

Results of the trial were recently reported in the *PLOS One journal.* "These are extremely exciting findings and indicate that vaccination (immunotherapy) may act synergistically with rescue chemotherapy to improve second remission duration and prolong overall survival," Mason said. "We are now working on a similar, second generation vaccine and have just initiated a second clinical trial to evaluate its effectiveness in preventing relapse following induction chemotherapy. The vaccine will be given every three weeks for a total of three times and then every two months thereafter." The trial is funded by the Canine Health Foundation and is actively recruiting patients at this time.

Teleromase Cancer Vaccine

One hallmark of cancer cells is limitless replication. Aged or damaged cells bypass apoptosis and continue to divide. (See apoptosis, page 13.) An enzyme called teleromase has been found to be overexpressed in human and animal cancer cells. Researchers theorize that it may be teleromase that causes or allows cells to bypass apoptosis—to continue uncontrolled division as cancer cells.

As part of a study to test this theory, a therapeutic vaccine treatment is available for dogs with lymphoma. It is targeted immunotherapy, which attacks canine teleromase, thus inhibiting the replicative ability of cancer cells and restricting further uncontrolled division.

The non-funded study is led by the veterinary research team of Dr. Joe Impellizeri, oncologist from Veterinary Oncology Services (VOS) in

Middletown, NY and Long Island, Dr. Luigi Aurisicchio from Takis Biotech in Rome, Italy and Dr. David Jemiolo from Vassar College. To date, VOS is the sole veterinary oncology center in the United States to offer the telomerase vaccine for canine and feline cancer patients. (Information at www.petcancerinformation.com)

As it happens, Dr. Impellizeri at was a member of Bullet's cancer team and has been keeping me up to date. According to Dr. Impellizeri (email April, 2014), published data supports longer survival for canine lymphoma patients when the vaccine is combined with standard of care chemotherapy. Dr. Impellizeri says,

> *"The future of oncology treatment in both people and animals will include targeted therapies such as telomerase. Immunotherapy is a marathon, not a sprint, and must be started as early as possible to allow the immune response to respond against the remaining cancer cells.*
> *Our goal, specifically in canine lymphoma patients, is to obtain clinical and molecular remission with standard of care (CHOP) chemotherapy and follow it with the teleromase vaccine as an additional mechanism to battle the cancer."*

October 27, 2015, Dr. Impellizeri emailed saying, "Laurie, the U.S. data has just been presented at the 2015 VCS conference. Data shows even better results than the initial European-published data, by exceeding the seventy-eight week median survival for combined standard lymphoma chemotherapy plus telomerase vaccine."

Vaccine Therapy for Dogs with Osteosarcoma

Also being evaluated by Dr. Joe Impellizeri at Veterinary Oncology Services (www.petcancerinformation.com), is a vaccine for dogs with osteosarcoma using the canine biomarker HER2/neu. The aim of this vaccine, given after surgery and with chemotherapy, is to eliminate remaining osteosarcoma cells. Dr. Impellizeri explains:

> *"If the dog's immune system is successfully stimulated by this vaccine, then it is expected that immune cells will find and eliminate any remaining cancer cells that have avoided standard chemotherapy.*

Furthermore, it is hoped that the immune system will develop a 'memory' of these cancer cells and will be able to prevent further osteosarcoma lesions from developing."

BMT for Dogs with Lymphoma

To start the Bone Marrow Transplant (BMT) or hematopoietic stem cell transplantation procedure, clean, cancer-free stem cells are extracted from the dog's bone marrow. If the stem cells are taken from the dog being treated, this is *autogenic* BMT. If they are taken from a donor dog, this is *allogenic* BMT.

Next, high doses of RTx are given to kill the dog's mature bone marrow cells. The dog's immune system is destroyed. Then, the dog remains in the clinic, in isolation, for about two weeks. This is necessary because without an immune system, any exposure to infection could be fatal.

During this time, the clean, cancer-free stem cells are reintroduced intravenously. When they begin to repopulate the marrow, engraftment takes place, and the cleansed marrow will again be able to produce new blood cells.

Dr. E. Donnall Thomas, at the Fred Hutchinson Cancer Research Center in Seattle, WA, used dogs as subjects to develop BMT as a cancer cure for humans. He began this work in 1955 in NY, continued at Seattle's Providence Hospital in 1963, and in 1975 moved his team to the Fred Hutchinson Cancer Research Center.

BMT is used to treat human leukemia with very good success. Human leukemia is no longer considered a terminal disease. Due to Dr. Thomas' work and thanks to the dogs that were used to develop the treatment, it is now considered a treatable disease. Dr. Thomas received the 1990 Nobel Prize in physiology or medicine for this work.

After approval was given for use of BMT for humans, the treatment was no longer available to dogs. That hardly seems fair! But at that time, veterinary oncology was not yet a booming business and pet owners were not ready to enlist their dogs for the treatment.

Recently, BMT was reintroduced into veterinary medicine. Dr. Edmund Sullivan is a veterinarian in Bellingham, WA, credited with doing one of the first nonexperimental marrow transplants for a dog. In 2004, he provided BMT for a Golden Retriever named Comet, who had T-cell lymphoma. Comet is celebrated as the first canine BMT success story. He survived another four years.

Because dogs had been instrumental in developing the treatment for humans, Dr. Sullivan said, "It's only fair that we now make this widely available as a treatment option for them [dogs] as well."

> *Bullet's diagnostic biopsy stated that he had late-stage lymphoma. He had the standard chemo protocol, a CHOP protocol very similar to the Modified Madison-Wisconsin Protocol. Bullet's first chemotherapy treatment achieved a remission. He completed the protocol and the remission lasted the rest of his natural life, more than four years. This was an exceptional survival. Exceptional, but not rare. There are many dogs that have exceptional survivals of three or four years after a CHOP protocol.*

Comet's was an exceptional survival. However, since Bullet and other dogs given a CHOP protocol without BMT survive for two, three or four years, it is possible that Comet would have as well.

Successful new treatments are published in the veterinary journals. The results for BMT are not, and several veterinarians have expressed to me that this raises suspicion about the treatment's success.

Veterinarians who offer it are promoting it heavily as a well established and successful treatment. While dog owners are aggressively recruited to allow BMT on their dogs with lymphoma, veterinary oncologists are still working to improve the dismal success rate. One of the primary proponents is Dr. Steven Suter VMD PhD ACVIM (Oncology), Assistant Professor-Medical Oncology, Medical Director: Canine Bone Marrow Transplant Unit, Dept. of Clinical Sciences, North Carolina State University College of Veterinary Medicine in Raleigh NC. Dr. Suter told me (email, 12/9/2011) that he was still making adjustments to the amount of irradiation and the amount of chemotherapy that should be given with the BMT protocol in order to improve the survival time.

In a news release from North Carolina State University College of Veterinary Medicine, Dr. Suter says, "While the survival rate with current treatments [chemotherapy] is extremely low—about 0 to 2 percent—the cure rate for dogs that have received a bone marrow transplant is at least 30 percent." Suter added, "The process itself is painless for dogs - the only thing they lose is a bit of body heat while the cells are being harvested."

This statement is misleading and simply untrue. First, it under-reports the success of chemotherapy alone, and exaggerates the success of BMT for dogs with lymphoma. Standard CHOP-based protocols have a published success rate for remission of over 90 percent and a median one-year survival of more than 300 days. Dr. Dave Ruslander, estimated the success rate of standard chemotherapy for dogs with lymphoma at 50 percent with a twelve- to eighteen-month survival, 35 percent with a two-year survival, and 5 to 10 percent with a four-year survival.

Second, the statement neglects to mention that the treatment is extremely selection-biased. While the standard chemo protocol is given to almost any dog with lymphoma, BMT is given only to dogs that have already achieved remission (thanks to chemo), are under a certain age, have no concurrent illnesses, and are strong and healthy. BMT is given only to the dogs that have the best chance of long-term survival regardless of the treatment protocol they are given. A better comparison would be dogs given a CHOP chemotherapy protocol who stayed in remission for two months, vs dogs given BMT.

Some dogs given BMT who die due to the rigors of the treatment might have survived a year or more if given the standard chemo protocol. BMT costs the owner between $10,000 and $21,000, whereas standard chemo costs between $3,000 and $6,000.

I asked Dr. Ruslander about BMT and he replied, "Bone marrow transplant … has resulted in increased survival times and overall cure rates in humans. This has not been proven in canine lymphoma, although we would expect it to be similar." He went on to say, "Morbidity, including possible infections and immune suppression, is moderate to high, and there is a chance of fatal infections in a moderate number of patients, but again data is somewhat lacking." (Email, 12/11/2012.)

I asked Dr. Alice Villalobos for an opinion about BMT for dogs. She said, "Expensive and risky, just as it is for humans. Most of the cases I have been familiar with did not get more time than those dogs given the standard protocols." (Email, 12/14/2012.)

▷ ***Nikki Vulin's BMT Story***
I'm a little bitter about BMT because the treatment failed to meet expectations for my Nikki. The science behind BMT may be sound but it is very risky.

Dogs have died because of the procedure itself. One poor dog, who looked very much like Nikki, had BMT. She never engrafted and she died at the hospital.

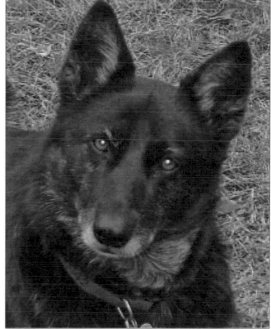

There is a very high risk of infection and bleeding while the white blood cell and platelet counts are low due to the irradiation.

Dr. Suter said to me that the dogs given BMT tend to see relapses at the eighteen-month mark. The veterinarians at Tufts University School of Veterinary Medicine told me that a lot of people choose euthanasia for their dog after the first relapse. If these statements are both true, I do not understand how a 30 percent cure rate could be possible.

Why did I choose BMT for Nikki? It was an emotional decision. I was told that this was a treatment option with a potential cure, and I just could not bring myself to deny my Nikki the chance to be cured. I wanted her to have a 30 percent chance at survival, rather than a 0 to 2 percent chance.

Nikki relapsed after nine months. I don't regret having done it because if I hadn't, I would have spent the rest of my life wondering "What if?" On the other hand, now I will always wonder how Nikki would have fared if she had just had chemo.

- Lillian Vulin, Shrewsbury, Massachusetts

Other Treatments and Therapies

Tumors release chemicals that stimulate the production of a new network of blood vessels. As a tumor forms, it creates its own network of vessels to provide the blood supply it will need to grow. This development is called *angio* (blood vessel) *genesis* (birth or beginning). In the absence of angiogenesis (without the blood supply provided by new blood vessels), tumors are unable to grow.

Antiangiogenesis

In *antiangiogenesis*, substances that inhibit the formation of new vessels are introduced in an attempt to cut off a tumor's blood supply and thereby kill the tumor.

Dr. Chand Khanna, DVM, PhD, DACVIM (oncology), president of the Animal Cancer Institute, has researched antiangiogenic agents. Dr. Khanna explains this treatment in the following excerpt from "Targeting the blood supply of cancer," Animal Clinical Investigation, LLC, 2002.

> *"Agents that inhibit new blood vessel formation or specifically target tumor-associated blood vessels represent a novel, potentially effective and nontoxic treatment for cancer. It is likely that these agents will provide the next major breakthrough in the management of pet animals and people with cancer."*

One famous antiangiogenesis success story involves a dog called Navy. Navy was treated with COX-2 inhibitors and anti-angiogenics. As of July 2002, Navy had maintained a sixteen-month remission without chemotherapy. This "cure" inspired new research into antiangiogenesis, although it has not been successfully and reliably repeated in other dogs.

Stories of spontaneous remissions and miracle cures are plentiful in pets and in humans. They lead to a flurry of excitement and a bonanza in sales of whatever treatment or supplements were given to the survivor.

It's possible that when spontaneous remission occurs, a random combination of therapies or a genetic anomaly is responsible. Occasionally, in other words, even a blind squirrel finds an acorn.

Radiation Therapy for Dogs with Lymphoma

Over the past two decades, there have been many efforts to find a way to use RTx for dogs with lymphoma. A variety of protocols have been used. One of the protocols was giving the dog two treatments of total-body irradiation (TBI) in addition to chemotherapy. Another was giving half-body irradiation (HBI) in addition to chemotherapy. To date, RTx for dogs with lymphoma has not improved survival times over a standard chemotherapy protocol such as the Modified Madison Wisconsin, or CHOP protocol.

Cryosurgery

In cryosurgery, liquid nitrogen or nitrous oxide is used to "freeze" the tumor rather than to surgically excise it. This method is used to treat cutaneous and subcutaneous tumors, tumors on the skin, eyelid, and perianal area, and oral tumors. Cryosurgery has found its place primarily with the holistic veterinary practitioner.

Relative to traditional surgery, cryosurgery is a shorter procedure with less trauma to the dog, and it is less costly. It is a good solution when an owner wants a superficial tumor or mass simply removed, without expectations of additional treatment.

If you will want to find out what type, stage, and/or grade cancer your dog has, a tissue sample should be removed for biopsy before the treatment is performed.

Tumor sites that should not be treated with cryosurgery include osteosarcoma of long bones, intranasal tumors, circumferential anus tumors, large mast cell tumors, and other large, aggressive tumors.

Photodynamic Therapy

Like cryotherapy and hyperthermia, this treatment exposes cancer cells to a stimulus in hopes that they will, as a result, become damaged and die. In photodynamic therapy (PDT), the stimulus is a three-way combination, including a photosensitizer (IV or topically) to make the tissue more responsive to the treatment; a light source; and oxygen, which is required to complete the photochemical oxidative process.

Dr. Dudley McCaw, DVM, ACVIM, wrote about photodynamic therapy in *Veterinary Oncology Secrets* (Hanely & Belfus, Inc, 2001). According to Dr.

McCaw, PDT has been used in veterinary medicine for transitional cell carcinoma and canine oral squamous cell carcinoma. In some countries, it has been approved for use in humans for lung, esophageal, bladder, and gastric cancers.

There's a potential for PDT treatment to benefit cancer patients in the future. Much is still unknown about exactly how it works and how to make it work more efficiently.

Alternative Therapies

There are several alternative therapies that might be helpful to add to your arsenal in your fight against your dog's cancer. They may or many not be recommended by your veterinarian, but they will not do any harm to your dog.

Acupuncture

Acupuncture does not cure or treat cancer, but can alleviate side effects during cancer treatment, support organs in need of fortification, and generally balance body systems and energy flow.

When Bullet was in remission from lymphoma for a few months, I asked our holistic vet Dr. Bea Ehrsam, DMV, about the advisability of giving him acupuncture. She recommended against it. She said that acupuncture can be a stimulator, and it's impossible to predict exactly what will be stimulated. Dr. Ehrsam said that she would rather not take a chance since Bullet was doing so well in remission.

Dr. Rodney Page, DVM, DACVIM (internal medicine; oncology), is the Director of Colorado State University's Flint Animal Cancer Center. Dr. Page says, "Of the current alternative therapies, I believe acupuncture has the most solid evidence of benefit for the relief of neurogenic or orthopedic pain developing from cancer."

Massage

Does your dog enjoy a massage? Who doesn't! Massage will soothe your dog, it will be a time for bonding, and it will benefit you as well. It may encourage circulation and healing (in both of you), and will allow you to discover new lumps or bumps early. When massaging a dog with cancer, the hand movements should travel away from the heart.

Synchronized Breathing

If your dog's breathing is labored, shallow, or uneven, lie next to him. The spoon position works well here. Synchronize your breathing to his and then very gradually shift your breathing to a deep, even pattern. You may hear your dog's breathing shift, trying to stay in time with yours. When you hear a deep, slow breath, a heavy sigh, a cleansing breath, your mission is accomplished.

Other

Myofascial release, Tellington TTouch®, Reiki, and other healing-touch techniques may encourage healing, circulation, and relaxation. Reports of efficacy vary and most if not all of the evidence that they have any effect is anecdotal.

> *While Bullet was having chemotherapy treatments, my friend Malea Barber provided distance Reiki treatments. I would lay down on the floor holding Bullet and I knew that at a certain time, Malea was going to send her treatment to him. At the appointed time, I almost always felt a marked change in his breathing. I felt his body relax completely. I don't know if the treatments played a part in keeping Bullet in remission, or in fighting his cancer, but do attest that it had a positive effect.*

Clinical Trials

Clinical trials are routinely conducted at schools of veterinary medicine, at large veterinary hospitals with specialty services, and at veterinary practices that participate in networks or collaborate with local hospitals.

Most clinical trials for chemotherapy are set up to test variations on a theme. None of the chemo drugs commonly used for dogs was discovered or developed in the past twenty years. Existing protocols are tweaked in an effort to improve the outcome—to compare the known success of an accepted protocol with the success of the same protocol when given over an abbreviated or extended time period, in different amounts, dosages, titration, combinations, and/or on a different schedule.

A "new treatment" that is actually still in clinical trial may be presented to you as the next new cure for the disease that your dog has. In order to complete the necessary step of recruiting subjects into a clinical trial, your veterinarian may misrepresent a trial to you as the up-and-coming cure for your dog's cancer.

If the allure of a clinical trial is that it may reveal a treatment that will be more effective than current treatments, or that it may be an amazing cure for cancer, this may not be the best reason to request enrollment. Almost all clinical trials prove in the end to be less effective than traditional treatment.

During the research and development phase, a treatment is given at various strengths to find the upper limit of what may be helpful and tolerated. It is given at lower strengths until the point is found at which it is no longer effective. Thus, treatments are tested in an effort to minimize toxicity and maximize efficacy. Some trials result in death from cancer (when a less potent treatment is tested to decrease toxicity), or in death from treatment (when a more potent treatment is tested to increase efficacy).

As much as you would like to believe that the new treatment offers survival, keep these things in mind before you offer your dog as a trial subject.

- ▶ Newly discovered drugs and therapies may be thrown out as a net to be tested as a possible treatment for many different types of cancer. If some success is found with one cancer, they say *"Let's try it on everything, and let's see what else it might help."*
- ▶ Only 5 percent of new agents investigated for cancer treatment will eventually prove to be successful and receive approval from the Food and Drug Administration.

   According to Dr. Cheryl London, veterinarian and cancer researcher at Ohio State University's Veterinary Medical Center, "About 80 percent of clinical trials fail in the early stages, and a little less than half fail in the later stages."

   According to CenterWatch, only about one out of every 50

drugs tested in animals is determined to be safe and effective enough to test in humans.

According to the Morris Animal Foundation website, "Clinical trials... can offer cutting-edge treatment, often at a reduced cost to the owner. Trials are scientific research designed to answer specific clinical questions, including whether the new experimental treatment has a therapeutic effect on the pet's disease, whether the new or experimental treatment is better than the current standard therapy and whether the procedure or treatment is well tolerated." To me, cutting-edge treatment means a new treatment that is effective against the disease. Not treatment that is being tested (on your pet) to find out if it will be effective or not.

▸ In some trials, funding is available to help owners manage the costs. A very good and fair offer will look something like this: "There is no fee to participate in this study. Once your dog is enrolled, costs associated with initial cancer staging and restaging three weeks after treatment, the study drug administration, monitoring, and treatment of any side effects are paid for by the study."

▸ Participants may be required to forgo other treatments that have documented success or to grant permission for an autopsy to be performed if your dog dies during the trial. Read the fine print!

Look to clinical trials when there is no traditional treatment available with a good success rate, or when budgetary constraints make other treatments impossible. If you discover a trial appropriate for your dog, ask your veterinarian to find out if he can participate in the trial and provide the treatment. Find current trials at www.vetcancertrials.org/studies.

10

What's Your Dog Eating?

Dogs have been domesticated for over 14,000 years, but the dog food industry has been around less than a century. Technology stepped in to save owners time—to make feeding as simple, tidy, and effortless as pouring pellets into a bowl. It's easier for us, but is it healthy for our pets?

Many commercially produced dog foods are comprised of poor quality ingredients that have been cooked at extremely high temperatures, thus destroying much or all the natural nutritional content. Nutrients listed on the product label are in the food only because they have been added back in as additives, after processing. If you wish to feed "dog food" to your dog with cancer, at least buy one with a low carbohydrate content.

There is an alternative! You can feed your dog "real" food—i.e., whole foods, human-grade foods, and unprocessed foods. More and more dog owners are choosing not to feed their pets canned or bagged food. You have probably heard the warning, *"Don't feed your pets table food—it will kill them!"* It may or may not, depending on what you eat!

I'm not suggesting that you feed your dog a diet of table scraps or serve him up a dish of whatever you and your family are having for breakfast, lunch, and dinner. I am suggesting that you roll up your sleeves and prepare for your dog a natural diet. Feeding a dog a natural or "wild-type" diet means providing him with a diet that mimics what a dog (or a wolf, with a nearly identical genetic makeup to the dog) eats in the wild.

The canid in the wild doesn't intentionally eat fruits and vegetables. He does, however, eat the stomach and intestines of his prey, which may contain partially digested fruits and vegetables. We can mimic this in a dog's diet by including fruits and vegetables that have been well cooked or pulverized in a food processor, to enable the dog's digestive system to extract the nutrients.

Wolf biologist L. David Mech says that the stomach of the prey is rarely eaten by the predator wolf. Nonetheless, most wild-type canine diets do include pulverized or steamed vegetables.

Raw and "Wild-Type" Diets

Preparing food for a dog is more involved than pouring kibble into a bowl, but it is much simpler, less time consuming and less expensive than you might think.

The meat in a truly wild diet comes from deer, caribou, mice, and other animals that are natural prey of the wolf. Muscle meat and organs, some cartilage, and bone of the prey animal are all consumed. What about preparation? The wild canine predator certainly does not build a fire and cook his kill. He eats it raw.

Many dog owners feed their not-so-wild dogs a wild-type diet with raw meat. This is still controversial among veterinarians. As might be expected, traditional veterinarians are generally against it and holistic veterinarians are for it.

The wild canine has a digestive tract and digestive acids that enable him to process, digest and ingest raw meat. Is the domestic canine suscep-tible to bacterium such as salmonella and E. coli? Some veterinarians feel that dogs are invulnerable to these "bugs," while others feel they are susceptible, and still others claim that the diet is safe so long as the food is frozen before serving.

If you change your dog's diet, do so gradually. This rule applies whether you are switching from store-bought food to prescription food, from kibble to home-cooked, or from home-cooked to raw. Mix one-quarter of the new diet with three-quarters of the old, for a week. Continue to increase the new, and decrease the old by one-quarter each week. At the end of the month, donate remaining cans or bags of food from your dog's old diet to your local shelter.

If any vomiting or diarrhea results while you are changing your dog's diet, return to the diet that was more agreeable to his digestive system. Some dogs simply don't tolerate raw food, and some owners don't feel comfortable serving it. Whether you choose to serve your dog store-bought food, or raw or cooked homemade food is a personal decision for you and your dog to make.

Bullet ate a raw diet, and to abolish any harmful bacteria that might be lurking, particularly in the meat, I always froze Bullet's food before serving. I prepared a month's worth of food for him at a time, one Sunday a month. I often tossed him tidbits of raw meat that had not yet been frozen. In more than three years, he never suffered any ill effects.

After two years in remission, Bullet developed a heart condition. To play it safe, I fed him a lightly cooked version of the same diet. I boiled, baked, or broiled the meat and steamed the vegetables.

The food that you make for your dog is full of fresh and natural nutrients, vitamins, and minerals—not the kind that are added into processed food after all of the natural ones have been destroyed during processing.

About Diet and Cancer

There has been extensive research toward understanding the relationship between nutrition and cancer. Much of what's known about the effect of diet on canine cancer is thanks to the research of Dr. Gregory K. Ogilvie, DVM, DACVIM (internal medicine and oncology).

Dr. Ogilvie's team and Hill's Pet Nutrition, Inc.® worked together to develop Hills® Prescription Diet® n/d® Canine. Studies have shown that dogs with lymphoma in chemotherapy and dogs with nasal or oral cancer in radiation therapy that eat n/d have a significantly longer survival rate than those who eat other commercially produced dog foods. Very possibly, dogs with any type of cancer would benefit from n/d; other cancers have simply not been tested.

Dietary guidelines for dogs with cancer are based on two important concepts. First, cancer cells readily metabolize carbohydrates. Second, cancer cells are unable to metabolize fats. The goal is to feed the patient, not the cancer.

Your objective is to include in your dog's diet what he is able to utilize (what his cancer cells are unable to utilize). And to withhold what the cancer cells are going to utilize, thus making its nutritional value unavailable to your dog.

The Canine Cancer Diet contains
low carbohydrates,
moderate protein, and
high Omega-3 fatty acids

A diet low in carbohydrates does not include foods that contain sugar or starch, such as fruits, grains, potatoes and some vegetables. Dog biscuits are usually high in carbohydrates. If you feel biscuits are essential to maintain your dog's quality of life, then choose one with a low carbohydrate content and limit the number of biscuits you give him per day.

A high-fat diet contains Omega-3 fatty acids. Flax seed oil, cod liver oil, and fish oil are at the top of this list. Flax seed oil has the highest Omega-3 fatty acid content, but also contains O-6 fatty acids. Actually, all of the fatty acids contain Omega-6. The most important factor to consider is the proportion of Omega-3s to Omega-6s. For a dog with cancer, we want the highest ratio of Omega-3s to Omega-6s.

When Omega-3 fatty acids are added nutritionally or as supplements, antioxidants should be given as well. Oils in a canine diet that provide Omega-3 fatty acids should not be heated. Whether you serve your dog cooked or raw food, the oils can be added into the final mixture and frozen, or added to individual meals when served.

There is an exception to the recommendation of adding Omega-3 fatty acids to the diet of a dog with cancer. Two veterinary oncologists have told me that the oils may actually protect cancer calls from irradiation and decrease the effectiveness of radiation therapy. If your dog is having radiation therapy, consult with your veterinarian to find out when it will be safe to begin adding fatty acids to the diet.

Some owners are not willing to, not capable of, or just don't have time to prepare a homemade diet for their dogs with cancer. Many of them feed their dogs Evo® by Natura Pet Products® because it is a high quality food with low carbohydrate content. Some of the Evo products contain as little as 12 percent carbohydrate content, from fruits and potatoes. In a diet for a dog with cancer, the carbohydrate content should not be more than 12 or 14 percent.

Most commercial dog food products do not print the carbohydrate content on the label. However, there is a nifty formula offered by dogfoodadvisor.com that will help you figure out the carbohydrate content of any dog food. Add up the protein, ash, fat, and water content percentages. Subtract that from 100, and you will have the approximate carbohydrate content.

L-Arginine is a helpful supplement for dogs with cancer. When a dog with cancer is fed commercial dog foods or a home made diet (other than n/d), L-Arginine should be added in as a supplement.

Who to Consult about Diet

Why not ask a veterinary oncologist? They are the experts in the diagnosis and treatment of cancer, but are generally not experts about the role diet and supplements play. We depend on them for their expertise in chemotherapy or surgery or radiation. We do not need to depend on them for information about diet and supplements.

Holistic veterinarians are the experts when it comes to diet and supplements. They are also knowledgeable about diet and supplements specifically for a dog with cancer.

> *After Bullet's chemotherapy protocol was completed, our wonderful Dr. Porzio moved to Canada. I wanted to line up an oncologist so that "just in case" Bullet came out of remission, I would know where to take him. I made an appointment with a local veterinary oncologist. In a twenty-minute session, the veterinarian spoke to me academically and pedantically about lymphoma remission and rescue protocols. She never looked at Bullet or touched him.*
>
> *When I said that Bullet ate a raw diet, she said that she would not provide treatment to him while on a raw diet. I told her that Bullet was on a raw diet for the entire seventy-five weeks that he was in chemo, with no problems. She didn't care, she would not treat him. Really? If Bullet did need treatment, and if I wanted to see this vet, I could easily have told her that he was eating kibble.*
>
> *I was also astounded that anyone could be in a room with Bullet and not be pulled in by his sweetness and his beauty. What kind of a person wouldn't have an irresistible urge to run their fingers through his luxurious coat and look into those icy blue eyes? And why would such a person choose to be a vet?*

Before Bullet was diagnosed, I fed him meat, whole grains, and vegetables in equal proportions (one-third each). Unlike Bullet's Cancer Diet, this diet contained carbohydrates. Although carbs have fallen out of favor, our cells—and our dogs' cells—need carbos to generate energy. Including carbohydrates also lowers the cost a homemade diet for a healthy dog. But after a diagnosis of cancer, we need to exclude the carbohydrates.

If you have a dog with cancer and a dog without cancer, you can prepare both at once, and make a few adjustments either before freezing or before feeding.

Prepare Bullet's Cancer Diet for both dogs, but without the oils. Also prepare three cups of grains (such as rice, cous cous or quinoa). At feeding time, add cooked grains to the dish for your healthy dog. Add additional oils to the dish that your cancer dog is waiting for.

Bullet's Cancer Diet

Quantities below are for one week of fine dining for an eighty-pound dog. By weight, the mix is about ¾ meat to ¼ vegetables. By volume it will look like half and half. Start with the ingredients list and quantities below, and then have fun making substitutions of various vegetables. You can base the ingredients list on what vegetables happen to be in your refrigerator.

Meat may be raw or cooked. Vegetables may be steamed or pulverized. Supplements that can be given with food can be added before serving.

Ingredients

Beef, chicken, or turkey	6 Lbs.
Tomatoes	4
Cabbage	¼ Lb.
Broccoli	¼ Lb.
Kale (dark green leaf)	¼ Lb.
Eggs	6
Tofu	¼ Lb.
Fatty acids (flax seed or fish oil)	10 Tbsp.
Hulled or milled flax seeds	2 Tbsp.

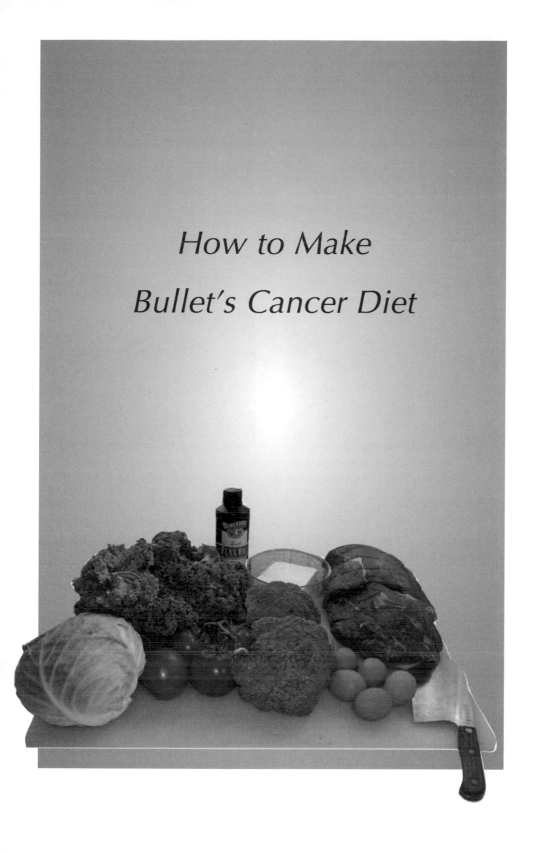

How to Make

Bullet's Cancer Diet

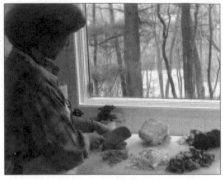

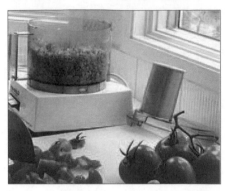

1 Chop broccoli, cabbage, kale and/or other green vegetables. Put through food processor.

2 Cut up tomatoes and run through food processor.

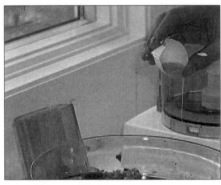

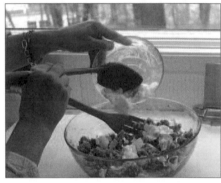

3 Add egg yolks. Drop whites and crumbled shells into another bowl and cook. Raw egg whites deplete biotin, which your dog needs.

4 Cook egg whites and crumbled shells on the stove or in a microwave until the egg-white is solid enough to cut with a fork.

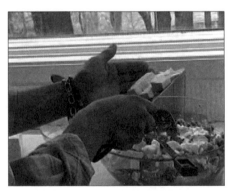

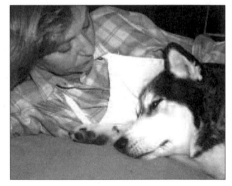

5 Tofu is a good source of protein. Cube and add tofu. Hand mix as though tossing a salad.

6 **Take a Break!** If your dog works as hard as Bullet did, he's exhausted by now. You can cover and refrigerate overnight if you want to finish tomorrow.

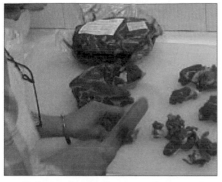

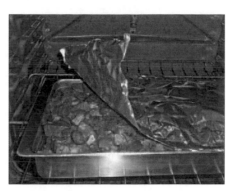

7 Cube meat into bite-sized pieces. Use beef, chicken, turkey or fish.
* If your dog picks out the meat and leaves the rest, use ground meat.

8 If you are cooking the contents, cook meat and vegetables now. Allow all to cool before proceeding.

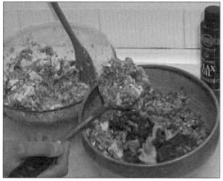

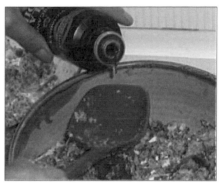

9 Combine all and mix like tossing a salad. Next you'll add Omega-3 fatty acids. Use flax seed, fish, salmon, cod liver or olive oil. I use flax seed oil most frequently.

10 Add at least 2 Tbs. of oil per pound of meat. I confess I don't measure the oils. I pour in as much as the meat will absorb.

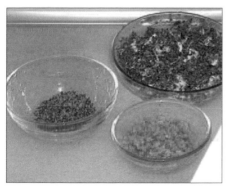

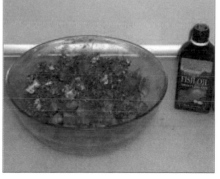

11 Add flax seeds. If they are not hulled or milled, run them through a coffee grinder.

12 Combine all and mix again. If you need to take a break, cover and refrigerate overnight.

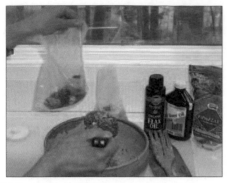

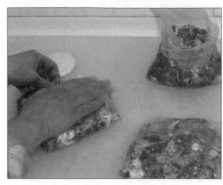

13 Scoop into plastic bags or freezer storage containers. Each bag or container should contain about three days of food.

14 Frozen food should not be exposed to air. After filling a bag, flatten it. Squeeze air out and pat it down flat.

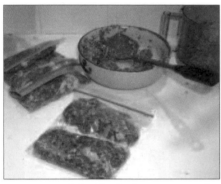

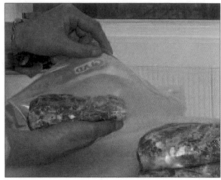

15 You can subdivide the bags per meal. If subdividing, use bags with zipper closures (not fold-over).

16 You can double-bag to keep bags free of air and the freezer free of drippings. Pack several small sandwich bags into a large air-tight bag.

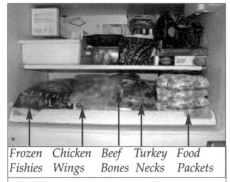

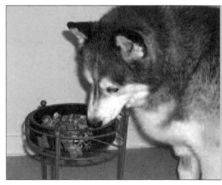

Frozen Fishies	Chicken Wings	Beef Bones	Turkey Necks	Food Packets

17 Freeze It! The bottom shelf of my freezer belonged to Bullet. Some dogs come running when they hear the sound of a can opener. Bullet came running to the sound of the freezer door opening.

18 **Thaw and serve!** At serving time add n/d, yogurt, cottage cheese and/or supplements and medications. Mix in water if your dog isn't drinking enough water.

Once a month, I purchased about twelve pounds of organic beef and about three pounds of vegetables, and spent a couple of hours preparing Bullet's food. This would last about three weeks. For the fourth week, I used something other than beef. I used chicken, turkey, or fish to give Bullet some variety.

If you are a mathematician, you will have noticed that the one-week diet above calls for six pounds of meat, but twice that amount lasted Bullet three weeks. This is not an error—Bullet was an "easy keep." He ate very little to maintain his weight. You'll need to watch your dog to see exactly what quantities he will need.

You and I need different quantities of food to maintain our weight and energy level. Even if we weigh exactly the same, our metabolisms and dietary requirements are unique. Likewise, each dog requires a different amount of food. Prescribed meal sizes should be used only as guidelines. While changing his diet, watch your dog's weight and energy level and adjust meal sizes accordingly.

I bought any cut of meat that the butcher had discounted, generally in slabs but occasionally ground. Bacteria can contaminate ground meat more quickly than unground meat. If you use ground meat, prepare, and freeze the meat as soon as possible.

Using ground meat shortens the preparation process appreciably. When I had limited time to get the diet prepared, I ordered ground beef. But the finished product was not as appealing to me. I liked to see the chunks of meat in the mix. For a dog who picks the meat out and leaves the rest, you do need to use ground meat so he will have to eat the entire meal.

My recipe was never the same from one batch to the next, but I always included beef, chicken or turkey (sometimes lamb, venison or fish). The core vegetables in Bullet's Cancer Diet are those high in vitamin C, low in sugar content, and considered important in a cancer-fighting diet. I included broccoli, cabbage, kale, and tomatoes. I sometimes made substitutions such as Brussels sprouts instead of Cabbage, Bok choy, spinach, or cauliflower. Use carrots and beets sparingly due to their high sugar content. Use cooked beans (lima, pinto, etc.) as well. Beans are another good ingredient for the diet, because they are high in protein.

The diet always includes an Omega-3 fatty acid, three or four vegetables, and eggs. Dr. Tina Aiken, DVM, at Pine Plains Veterinary Hospital in

Pine Plains, NY, helped me to create Bullet's diet. She recommended that I also include organ meat and ground bone.

There isn't any one food or combination of foods that you can feed your dog every time he eats, and be confident that you're giving him the best foods to fight cancer. Flexibility, variety, and rotation are important.

One benefit of feeding your dog a homemade diet rather than processed food is that he will be eating whole foods rather than processed foods. You will feel a connection to your dog when you place his bowl in front of him full of the food you prepared with your own two hands, and with the important ingredient of your love.

Another benefit is that it's easy to provide variety. You may be comfortable finding a diet that your dog likes and sticking to that. I had fun varying the ingredients and I felt that the variety kept Bullet more interested in eating his food.

After mixing the ingredients, I scooped the food into freezer bags or containers and placed these in the freezer. During the month, I thawed one bag in the refrigerator, and when Bullet ate the last meal from that bag, I rotated a new bag down from the freezer to the refrigerator.

When my schedule didn't allow for the full preparation routine, I prepared the diet piece-meal. I combined the meat and oils in containers and froze these. When I had time, I prepared the veggies and other ingredients in another container and froze them. At mealtime, I combined the two components. Then, when I served Bully his meals, I used two containers of thawed food instead of just one.

Bullet had virtually no carbohydrates in his diet for two solid years, with the exception of the "pound cake and pills combo," two dog biscuits daily, and the carbohydrate content in low-sugar vegetables. He had no grains, pasta, potatoes, bread, or cereal.

I honestly didn't think Bullet would live long enough to suffer negative consequences of a carbohydrate-deficient diet. I was wrong. About three years after remission, I reintroduced carbs into his diet, and he absolutely devoured them as though on some level he knew he'd been deprived of carbohydrates. Every night before bed, we each had a bowl of oatmeal.

You can make a delicious gravy to entice your dog to eat all of his food. After de-boning, put the bones in a pot of water. Cover and set to a low boil for a couple of hours. After they cool, remove the bones to capture the gravy. If you cook the meat, save the gravy.

Freeze gravy in containers and then thaw as needed to pour over your dog's meals, or add it to the portions you are going to freeze.

You can add kibble to the home made diet. This will accomplish two things. It makes the diet less expensive to prepare, and it will save you time. The batch of food you prepared will last longer when you add kibble to each meal.

Water

Dehydration can result from repeated vomiting or diarrhea, and can become dangerous. Monitor your dog's water intake and periodically check for dehydration (see page 134). Call your veterinarian right away if you suspect that he is dehydrated.

When Bullet was diagnosed, a nutritionist told me that although eating organic food and drinking filtered water may not be necessary for every one, they are essential when working to beat cancer. I was skeptical at the time, but her words have stayed with me, and now, years later, ring true.

In most areas of the country, tap water is shown in periodic studies to be potable, or safe to drink, with acceptable levels of toxins. "Allowable" levels of impurities in water may be tolerated by a dog or person with a healthy immune system, but for a cancer patient, filtered water is a must.

The simplest method of providing your dog with filtered water is to purchase a counter top filter and place it right over your dog's water bowl. Just open the spigot and fill the bowl. This is the most economical way of providing filtered water.

A more sophisticated (and expensive) method is installing a whole-house water filter. A state-of-the-art system would include a reverse osmosis filter that feeds into a spout at the kitchen sink. If you're considering installing a water filtration system, add to the "pro" column that the whole family will benefit! For homeowners, a good filtration system is a good investment and an attractive asset when you sell your house.

While at the Foster Hospital for Small Animals at Tufts with Bullet, I met a man called Michael Penney and his beautiful dog Hobbes. Hobbes had lymphoma and he was experiencing dehydration. Michael came up with an inventive method of increasing Hobbes's fluid intake. If your dog is dehydrated due to vomiting or diarrhea, or if you feel he's not drinking enough fluid, try Michael's solution:

- Mix gelatin (or pectin) with water per box directions
- Boil lean beef, chicken, or turkey in a small amount of water to make a concentrated broth
- Add broth to gelatin and let cool
- Pour into ice cube trays and place trays in the freezer

Your dog may eat the solidly frozen cubes right out of freezer, or may prefer to let them thaw and drink the liquid. "Meat-Jell-O" helped to get Hobbes to drink when he was reluctant to, and provided a bit of nutrition as well. *(Printed with permission of Michael E. Penney, Holliston, MA)*

Don't Forget the Treats

Most commercially produced dog treats are high in carbohydrates and are not on the "approved" list for our cancer dogs' consumption. Still, our cancer pups should certainly not be deprived of yummies! Quality of life includes being rewarded for good behavior and, in my book, survival is very good behavior indeed! We simply need to be creative. We need to find the treats that are good for our pups fighting cancer, and that they love to receive.

Try these cancer-healthy treats on your dog. If he doesn't biet, try anything you can think of that he might like without any sugar or starch.

- Plain, organic yogurt
- Cooked turkey or chicken meat, diced
- Raw, chopped vegetables. Try broccoli or string beans. Especially good for dogs who like crunchy treats.
- "Cheese bones." These are easy to prepare. Just press a slice of cheese into the end of a hollowed out, marrowless beef bone. A cheese bone will keep a dog busy for a while, is refillable and dishwasher-safe.

Frozen Treats

Bullet loved all of the following treats, and he ate them raw-frozen. Those marked "must be raw!" can have very serious or fatal consequences if served after being cooked. You can serve them frozen or thawed, but never cooked.

- Hill's n/d® (slide out of can, cube or slice, and freeze)
- Whiting or Pollock fillets; smelts
- Chicken hearts
- Beef bones (soup bones)—must be raw!
- Whole chicken wings—must be raw!
- Turkey necks—must be raw!

The items in this list that aren't followed by the note "must be raw" can be served cooked or frozen … but if cooked, they seem more like food items than treats, don't they?

Give Bullet's "Frozen Fishies" a try with your dog. They're the best dog treat ever, bar none. They are extremely healthy, they're simple and fun, and most dogs love them. They even get the back of a dog's teeth clean, where most of us don't manage to reach with the toothbrush. "Frozen Fishies" provide exercise for your dog's teeth and jaws! Frozen Fishies are simply the perfect dog treat.

See if your dog loves Bullet's "Frozen Fishies" as much as Bullet did. If he eats them immediately, you've got a winner. If not, you can cook them up for your own dinner!

Bullet's Treats
- Raw, frozen Whiting or Pollock fillet (frozen smelts for small dogs)
- Raw, frozen chicken wings or necks
- Raw, frozen chicken hearts
- Raw frozen beef bone with marrow
- "Cheese bones" (press cheese into a hollow raw beef bone; dishwasher-safe)
- Plain, organic yogurt
- Chopped up raw broccoli or string beans

Frozen Fishies!

When a dog in cancer treatment stops eating, there is cause for concern. Reversing the "not eating" state of affairs is of the utmost importance, even at the expense of breaking the cancer-diet rules. If your dog will not eat the foods recommended for cancer patients, get him to eat foods that are not recommended. Try deli meat, baby food, cat food, or oatmeal. Try anything and everything until you find the thing that he will eat.

During Bullet's first "flat out" episode, he stopped eating and showed no interest in food. He'd always been a chunky guy, so I didn't panic at first. I checked his temperature, and it was within the normal range. I thought Bullet was nauseous—a common chemotherapy side effect—so I gave him anti-nausea supplements, with no effect.

After several days passed and Bullet had not eaten anything at all, I became alarmed. I was now determined to get him to eat. I held bits of meat to his lips, trying to push the limp things into his mouth, with no success. I tried warming up the food, but he turned his head as though nauseated. After many attempts, I finally found success.

Siberian huskies are Northern dogs, sled dogs, happy eaters of frozen seal meat and the like. This mental image, combined with the realization that frozen food has little or no taste or smell and thus might be more palatable to a nauseous dog, prompted me to attempt the following:

I bought a bag of frozen smelt. I withdrew one and held its pointed tail in the corner of Bullet's mouth, poised to give a gentle push when his jaws opened. I applied only gentle pressure … and waited. Eventually, Bullet's jaws opened slightly and I pushed gently and waited. Lo and behold, just when my fingers were about to become completely numb, a chewing reaction began!

For a few days, I periodically offered Bullet food in a bowl or out of my hand. He was not planning to eat on his own, so I resorted to the "Frozen Fishies" method. After perhaps a week, when his gastrointestinal chemotherapy side effects diminished, the not-eating came to an end and Bullet returned to his normal eating habits.

If your dog isn't eating and you use the "Frozen Fishies" method, be patient and get comfortable! It may take some time for his chewing reaction to kick in. If he tries to push the fish out of his mouth with his tongue, gently replace it in the corner of his mouth. He may become ticked off at your efforts—in this case, of course, stop trying. We hope that he will instead become tired of pushing it out and let it rest there. Eventually, you will see a reflexive chewing action begin.

"Frozen Fishies" saved the day many times during Bullet's cancer treatment. After his appetite returned, he continued to eat "Frozen Fishies." I bought bags of Whiting and Pollock fillets, labeled "dressed fillets," in the frozen-fish section of the supermarket. They are not breaded and there's no sauce—just fish meat with no head, skin, or bones, ready to serve.

Bullet ate a "Frozen Fishies" every single day from that time forward, as have all of my dogs since then. I would toss a fish straight from the freezer onto the porch and Bullet would run after it, bark at it, toss it in the air, and then consume it happily.

If your dog likes "Frozen Fishies," toss a fillet straight from the freezer onto the porch or into the pen. No dishes to clean, nothing to mix, no muss, no fuss! I even toss them into the living room sometimes. So long as your dog eats the fillet while it's still frozen, there will be no fish residue or odor on the floor. Not so, however, for his breath! If you like to give your dog kisses, wait a while after he eats his Frozen Fishies, or give his teeth a good brushing before your next smooch.

11

What Else Can You Do?

Y ou decided on a medical plan. Now you ask, *"What else can I do?"* It's time to add supplements to your home-care regimen. Supplements and remedies can help to protect your dog from the ravages of chemotherapy, radiation, or surgery. And supplements can be used to fight cancer. The supplements that claim to fight cancer are, for the most part, unproven. Your selection process will therefore be largely intuition and guesswork.

Most veterinary oncologists do not recommend supplements for their canine patients. Some tell the dog owners to withhold antioxidants, amino acids, immune system boosters, etc., while a dog is in treatment. They may say that the supplements will lower the chance of treatment success.

The holistic veterinarian is the best source of information about supplements and their use for dogs with cancer, although they may not have cutting-edge information about chemotherapy protocols. Veterinary oncologists are the best source of information about chemo protocols although may not have cutting-edge information about diet and supplements.

A Labrador Retriever named Buddy appeared at the ACVIM's twenty-first annual forum in 2003. At that time he was nine and a half years old and had maintained a six-year remission from lymphoma. Dr. Marlene Hauck, DVM, PhD, assistant professor of oncology at North Carolina State University College of Veterinary Medicine, was Buddy's oncologist. I interviewed Dr. Hauck and learned that Buddy received the standard chemo protocol for lymphoma. She said that Buddy was fed "normal dog food" and did not receive any supplements or alternative treatments. And yet, Buddy survived more than six years after his diagnosis.

Despite Buddy's longevity without the benefit of dietary and supplemental therapies, many who have a dog with cancer want to cover all the bases, "just in case" the supplements actually might give their dogs a better chance at survival.

Give your dog supplements to support his fight against cancer and to aid and enhance medical treatment, but don't underestimate the power of supplements. You do not want to over-supplement. After all, pharmaceutical drugs do not come from another planet. Usually prescription drugs are formulated using the same elements that are in the supplements you will find in a health food store.

If a supplement can enhance a physiological or biochemical process, it can also over-enhance it. If a supplement can suppress a process, it can also suppress it too much.

Supplements are not harmless.
They should not be thrown together mindlessly.
Don't give your dog every supplement you hear about!

Be fluid and flexible in your choices so that you can do each day what's best for your dog according to his current status and needs. From time to time, you might want to add in a new supplement and/or omit one that you feel is less likely to be helping your dog fight cancer.

Few supplements, if any, have been tested sufficiently to inspire any certainty of efficacy. Most have been tested on a group of ten or twenty dogs without a control group and under conditions that are more anecdotal than scientific. The lack of testing is in large part due to the astronomical costs involved in performing the extensive testing required for FDA approval. Not many manufacturers of alternative health products can finance the testing and approval process.

The testing that has been done for most of the supplements is usually done without the controls necessary to qualify as FDA-level testing and the detailed results of the tests are not provided. The number of dogs in the test group may have been very small; dosages and frequencies might not be adequately controlled from one dog to another; and/or the testing was not conducted in a scientific manner.

There is always lots of anecdotal information about the success of a cancer-fighting supplement. You probably would not purchase one that doesn't include a testimonial about how it helped someone's dog. There may be a testimonial by a veterinarian. Some of the people quoted may have a monetary investment in the product.

Don't Blow a Fuse!

You will hear and read about many alternative treatments for cancer. There's an endless list of pills, gel caps, capsules, powders, tinctures, and teas that allegedly fight or cure cancer. Some may offer benefits and others may not help at all. You will probably be tempted to use all of them. Don't! You'll spend a great deal of money, become overwhelmed, and traumatize your dog with constant pilling.

I understand that you want to do everything you can to help your dog survive cancer. When you hear of a supplement that is said to fight cancer in dogs, you will want to go buy it and give your dog lots of it. Then you will read about or hear of another and another—there are hundreds, if not thousands. You will want to get those too, and lots of them!

Take a breath! Make an effort to choose supplements wisely and logically. There is no dog owner who has done *everything* that can be done for their cancer dog. It is not possible to provide every medical treatment, supplement, and alternative treatment.

I help owners develop home care plans for their dogs with cancer. Several times, I have received a list of fifty supplements and remedies they are using. The owner always seems proud of the size of the list. It is not true that the more supplements you give, the better chance your dog has of beating cancer. It's not true that giving your dog a hundred supplements is an indication that you love him more.

Don't let supplements wipe out your savings account. Don't blow a fuse keeping straight which to give when, how many times a day, with food or without. Don't exhaust and irritate your dog with constant supplementation. Begin with a few supplements you believe will be effective. When you learn from a reliable source of a new supplement that fights cancer, add it to your list and omit those you believe are less effective.

Instead of spending countless hours searching for more supplements to add, spend more quality time with your dog. Your dog would much rather play with you or lay his head on your lap, than watch you count pills, and click keys on your computer. Spending quality time with your dog does not include the time you spend researching, organizing supplements on a shelf, cutting up pills, making lists or feeding capsules and pills to him.

After Bullet was diagnosed with lymphoma, my kitchen counter was strewn with bottles containing his supplements. Each bottle was wrapped with a strip of masking tape with instructions written on it. BID, TID, with food, orally, alone, TID two days before chemo to two days after, BID not before or after chemo, etc.

I would venture into the kitchen several times a day, scan the array of bottles, vials, and powders and feel overwhelmed. Gradually, I eliminated some that I felt were superfluous, to narrow the list down to a reasonable size and to keep it current and dynamic.

Many dogs become reluctant to eat when they're ill, whether the illness is due to cancer, chemotherapy, or some other unrelated cause. If your dog is "off his foods" and you are working hard just to get some nutrition and essential medications into him, put aside any supplements that aren't working to heal his immediate condition until he is feeling better. Basic nutrition and the medications known to be effective are far more essential than the supplements that may or may not be effective.

Speak to your veterinarian and other cancer dog owners. If your veterinarian isn't up to speed on supplements (many are not), find a holistic veterinarian to consult in person or by phone.

After you decide on a list of supplements that you want to include in your regimen, you can comparison-shop for the best prices at a health food store and on the Internet. Some supplement products vary in quality from one manufacturer to another. Through companies such as Consumerlab.com, research the relative quality of supplements as produced by various manufacturers.

Vitamins and Minerals

Vitamins and minerals are fundamental to any dog's diet. When a dog is combating cancer, they are essential. In *Natural Health Bible for Dogs & Cats*, Dr. Shawn Messonnier, DVM states, "Studies demonstrate that both people and pets with inadequate nutrition cannot metabolize chemotherapy drugs adequately… This makes proper diet and nutritional supplementation an important part of cancer therapy."

General Guidelines

▸ Vitamins A, C, D, E, and K, and beta-carotene are important supplements for cancer patients because of their antioxidant properties.

▸ Vitamin A in combination with beta-carotene may benefit patients who are undergoing chemotherapy, surgery, or radiation therapy for cancer.

▸ Vitamin E is thought to protect against the ill effects of the chemotherapy agent doxorubicin while enhancing its effectiveness. Ask your veterinarian for the proper dosage of this vitamin.

▸ Zinc and magnesium may be helpful in the fight against cancer.

▸ If your dog is predominantly or fully a particular breed, ask your veterinarian if there are any deficiencies typical to that breed. For example, Siberian huskies tend to be zinc deficient.

Supplements

When you hear about a supplement that piques your interest, read up on it. Talk to veterinarians, other cancer-dog owners, and people who have used the supplement. Don't forget to search the net. Pose the question in an online support group for people who have a dog with cancer. After collecting your data, choose a group of supplements that you believe in. Remember, you can revise this list at any time.

Consult your veterinary oncologist, your holistic veterinarian, and/or your health store advisor to establish which supplements to give your dog and in what amounts. The following is not a comprehensive list.

Omega-3 Fatty Acids

As discussed earlier, Omega-3 fatty acids play an important role in fighting cancer. These supplements may be considered a part of the diet rather than supplements. If you do not feed your dog Bullet's Cancer Diet, be sure to provide your dog with Omega-3 fatty acids, either as part of his diet or as supplements. If your dog is being given radiation treatments, check with your vet. You may need to wait until treatments are completed before providing Omega-3 fatty acids.

Immune System and NK Cell Boosters

Some chemotherapy protocols are highly immunosuppressive. There are varying theories about the wisdom of using antioxidants to boost the immune system when medical treatment is designed to suppress it. Discuss this with your veterinarian or veterinary oncologist before you add immune boosters to your dog's regimen.

Many supplements claim to boost NK cell (natural killer cell) activity and/or production. NK cells attack other cells that are unwanted invaders, such as cancer cells. When cancer is present and a dog's NK cells are fighting an ever-growing army of cancer cells, the supply of NK cells may be depleted. Any cancer patient will benefit from increased NK cells. Here are some of the high-quality immune boosters to include in a home care regimen for a dog with cancer.

> ▶ K9-Immunity™ from Aloha Medicinals: A powerful immunomodulator containing nearly two hundred immunomodulator compounds.
> ▶ Agaricus Bio, from Atlas World USA, Inc: Enhances activity of macrophages that destroy or delay the proliferation of damaged cells.
> ▶ Astragalus: Available in capsules, tinctures, extracts, and ground or sliced root. Boosts the immune system and acts as a natural anti-inflammatory.
> ▶ IP-6: An NK (natural killer) cell booster that is formulated from rice, containing inositol hexaphosphate. Some formulas add maitake and cat's claw as well.

Antioxidants

Many vitamins, minerals, and herbs benefit cancer dogs because of their antioxidant properties. Antioxidants turn free radicals (cells that are missing one electron) into healthy cells by adding the missing electron. Free radicals are precursors of cancer cells. They are likely to become cancer cells if they are not converted into healthy cells through the addition of that missing electron.

Some veterinarians believe that antioxidants are counterproductive to chemotherapy. An article in *Alternative Therapies in Health and Medicine*

(Jan-Feb 2013) is titled "Antioxidants and Other Nutrients Do Not Interfere with Chemotherapy or Radiation Therapy and Can Increase Kill and Increase Survival, Part 1." The article states:

"Since the 1970s, 280 peer-reviewed in vitro and in vivo studies, including 50 human studies involving 8,521 patients, 5,081 of whom were given nutrients, have consistently shown that non-prescription antioxidants and other nutrients do not interfere with therapeutic modalities for cancer. Furthermore, they enhance the killing of thera-peutic modalities for cancer, decrease their side effects, and protect normal tissue. In 15 human studies, 3,738 patients who took non-prescription antioxidants and other nutrients actually had increased survival."

An article in *Integrative Cancer Therapies* (2007 Sep; 6(3):281-92) titled "Do Antioxidants Interfere with Radiation Therapy for Cancer?" states,

"Although further studies are needed, the preponderance of evidence supports a provisional conclusion that dietary antioxidants do not conflict with the use of radiotherapy in the treatment of a wide variety of cancers and may significantly mitigate adverse effects of treatment."

Studies show that antioxidants are not only safe, but are beneficial to dogs in chemotherapy. They may even enhance the effects of chemotherapy drugs. If you are not convinced, consult a holistic veterinarian to ensure that your dog is on the best antioxidant supplements to complement his medical treatment, his other supplements, and his nutritional intake.

Many antioxidants have (claim to have) curative or protective effects on a particular organ or system. These are noted below in parentheses.

- ▶ Vitamins A, C, D, E, and K, beta-carotene, and selenium.
- ▶ Black currant: Anti-inflammatory properties. (Skin)
- ▶ Cordyceps: Oxygenates the system. Not used before surgery or with anticoagulants. (Immune booster; kidneys; lungs)
- ▶ Coenzyme Q10: Can cause nausea at high doses. (Heart function; gum health)

- Curcumin (found in turmeric): Anti-inflammatory properties. (Heart function)
- Germanium sesquioxide: Oxygenates and dehydrogenates the blood. Give on alternate weeks—one week on, one week off. (Heart, lungs)
- Glutathione: An amino acid. Reduces damage to kidneys if used with chemotherapy agent cisplatin. Minimizes diarrhea when used with radiation therapy. (Immune system)
- Green tea extract: Protective against the effects of radiation therapy.
- Hawthorn: Improves heart function.
- Pycnogenol®: Pine bark extract with bioflavonoids. (Heart function; circulation)
- Quercetin: An antioxidant bioflavonoid. May enhance the effect of chemotherapy, radiation therapy, and hyperthermia. (Allergies; asthma)

Cancer Formulas
- Artemisinin: A Chinese herb that has killed cancer cells in a test tube.
- Poly-MVA™ (Polydox): A palladium lipoic complex (LaPd) and DNA reductase. May replenish nutrients depleted during chemo and radiation therapy.
- Transfer factors: Stimulate immune system function by enhancing the function of lymphocytes called T-helper cells.
- Essiac® tea: Burdock root, sheep sorrel, slippery elm bark, and Turkey rhubarb root. Acts as an antitumor antioxidant and immunostimulant.
- Hoxsey Cancer Formula: Berberine and other herbs. Cytotoxic, immunostimulating.
- Pau D'Arco and cat's claw: anticancer herbs. Alternate weekly rather than giving both together.
- Seacure®: biologically hydrolyzed whitefish. Protein supplement with many benefits. May alleviate chemotherapy side effects.
- Vacustatin: Angiogenesis inhibitor; antitumor agents. With PGM (proteoglycan mixture), from convolvulus arvensis (bindweed).

Organ Support

Chemotherapy and radiation are can damage body tissues including the digestive tract, kidneys, and liver. You can provide supplements that may protect these organs and systems as follows.

Gastrointestinal: L-Glutamine

Glutamine is an amino acid. It may be the most important supplement to give a dog in chemotherapy, to protect the lining of the small intestine. I have not found a canine study to support this statement, but *GUT Journal* issue 48:28-33 states, "A double-blind, placebo-controlled trial of 70 people undergoing chemotherapy... found that glutamine at a dose of 18 g daily improved intestinal function and structure, and reduced the need for antidiarrheal drugs."

For dogs in radiation therapy, *GUT Journal* Vol 35 Issue 1 says, "Comparison of diets with and without the added glutamine showed significant protection of the intestine from radiation injury."

For dogs having surgery, *The Annals of Surgery* v.227(2); Feb 1998 states, "We confirm the beneficial effects of Gln [glutamine]...on nitrogen economy, maintenance of plasma Gln concentration, lymphocyte recovery, cysteinyl-leukotriene generation, and shortened hospital stay in surgical patients.

Do not give your dog glutamine if he is taking anti-seizure medication. A ConsumerLab.com article states, "...because many anti-epilepsy drugs work by blocking glutamate stimulation in the brain, high dosages of glutamine might conceivably overwhelm these drugs and pose a risk."

Gastrointestinal: Acidophilus and Bifidus

These are good bacteria in the stomach that can be destroyed by chemotherapy. Provide acidophilus and bifidus in supplement form or add plain, organic yogurt with active cultures to your dog's daily diet.

Colon

Psyllium husks powder adds fiber to the diet, to cleanse the colon. Use only after discussing with your veterinarian.

Kidneys

Digestive enzymes such as ProZyme® ; Vitamin C.

Liver

Milk thistle detoxifies the liver. Give one-quarter tsp. twice a day starting several days after treatment, for about three days. My herbalist sent me wild-crafted milk thistle seeds with instructions to grind them in my coffee grinder and add to Bullet's "pound cake and pill mix."

SAMe is protective of the liver and has many other benefits.

Denamarin®: Contains SAMe (S-Adenosylmethionine) and milk thistle (silybin-phosphatidylcholine).

L-Arginine is an amino acid helpful in liver disease, heart disease, and cancer. It is included in n/d food. If you're not using n/d, provide L-Arginine as a supplement. The Mayo Clinic finds that "Early human studies suggest that arginine supplements may benefit people undergoing chemotherapy."

Heart

L-Carnitine may offer some protection for the heart particularly important when a dog is having treatment with Adriamycin.

Supplements with Antibiotic Properties

Tell your veterinarian about any supplements below that your dog is taking, before accepting a prescription for antibiotics.

▸ Bovine colostrum, a substance produced by a cow just prior to the production of mother's milk. It has powerful antibiotic properties. Available in powder or in encapsulated form.
▸ Echinacea defends primarily against upper respiratory infections.
▸ Goldenseal protects respiratory and digestive systems. This has antibiotic properties and stimulates the immune system.

Bullet's Supplements

Shortly after Bullet's diagnosis, I left an appointment with a holistic veterinarian with a bag full of bottles, vials, and boxes and with very little understanding of what they were or how they worked. As I gathered knowledge about the supplements, I fine-tuned his regimen many times. The supplements that I consider to be most important for a cancer dog (in addition to Vitamins E, C, B complex, and a multi-vitamin) are named below. If you use these, determine the correct quantities for your dog.

I found dried astragalus root at an herbalist's shop. Slices of the root resemble tongue depressors and can be steeped in soup, stew, or in a cup of tea. One day, a slice fell to the floor on its way to my teacup, and Bullet attacked it! He tossed it in the air, chased it, and devoured it entirely. I added it to my list of Bullet's treats, and also often sprinkled a three-finger pinch of shredded astragalus root onto his meals.

At times, Bullet ate astragalus eagerly and at other times showed no interest. According to my herbalist, he was self-medicating. He ate it when his system required it.

Supplements given to Bullet
- ▸ Antioxidants: cordyceps, CoQ10, germanium, quercetin, pycnogenol. I gave Bullet two or three different antioxidants at a time, in rotation. When I ran out of one, I incorporated a different one into his home-care regimen in its place. (Also vitamins C and E).
- ▸ Bovine colostrum: I gave this to Bullet as needed, whenever he had diarrhea and particularly when his stools contained blood. This is a natural antibiotic with many additional immune boosting benefits. It is collected in the first six hours after calving.
- ▸ Cancer formula: I rotated a variety of herbal concoctions claiming to fight cancer. Some of these were store-bought and others were prepared by my herbalist. Again, I attempted to cover all the bases.
- ▸ IP-6: Immune booster and NK cell booster Inositol hexaphosphate. About 800mg. twice a day.
- ▸ L-Arginine: 500 mg. twice a day. This is thought to be essential in fighting cancer.
- ▸ L-Glutamine: This is the most important supplement for any dog having chemotherapy treatment. I prefer the powdered version to capsules. It tastes slightly sweet, and packing it in a capsule is

unnecessary. I gave Bullet 1 tsp. of glutamine twice daily through-out his cancer treatment. I doubled the dose a few days before chemotherapy and for several days after. When he had any diges-tive or excretory problems, I tripled the dose.

▸ Poly-MVA®: At least 2ml two times a day, up to 4ml three times a day. Rub a few drops into any suspicious lumps or bumps. Poly-MVA can be given intravenously as well.

Contains minerals, B complex vitamins, palladium, amino acids and lipoic acid. Lipoic acid-palladium complex may alter the electrical charge of DNA molecules to help repair damaged DNA and cause cancer cells to self-destruct (see apoptosis, page 13).

Veterinary oncologist Dr. Gregory Ogilvie administers Poly-MVA for Pets as part of a cancer protocol for dogs.

▸ ProZyme®: I gave Bullet about 2 tsp. of this digestive enzyme in his food when he was having nausea, vomiting, or diarrhea.

▸ Wobenzym: Metabolic anti-inflammatory and immune support.

12

Whole Health Issues for Dogs with Cancer

Imagine that your dog survives cancer for six months or a year and your veterinarian finds that his teeth are in need of extensive dentistry. Most dental work requires anesthesia and involves a chance of infection—two things that any dog would be better off without, but particularly a dog that is fighting cancer. It's important to remember that health and medical issues are no less likely to occur to your dog than they are to a dog without cancer.

Keep your dog in tip-top condition while he is fighting cancer. Any neglected health issue can lead to unnecessary complications. Vitamin and mineral deficiencies can undermine any dog's strength. For a dog with cancer, the repercussions can be more severe and more difficult to resolve.

The emotional upheaval of finding that your dog has cancer, combined with the logistical complexities of providing cancer treatment, can be overwhelming. Depending on the complexity of your dog's cancer treatment and home-care plan, you may have your hands full. Incidentals such as bathing, grooming, and brushing his teeth may fall by the wayside.

The home-care tasks directly related to cancer will become routine before long and will require less of your time. Once this occurs, it's very important to reinstate a sound whole-health home-care program. Elderly folk quip, "If I knew I was going to live so long, I would have taken better care of myself!" Let's be optimistic and believe that your dog will live long enough, despite cancer, to benefit from your continued attention to his whole health.

During the course of cancer treatment, your dog may be immunosuppressed and therefore less able to ward off illness. When any secondary or unrelated health problem arises, find out what the treatment options are. Any veterinarians or specialists that you see should be aware of your dog's cancer status. The standard treatment for a particular illness may not be appropriate for a dog that also has cancer.

If a secondary illness occurs, contact all of your cancer team members to ask for their recommendation. Consider all treatment options offered by all factions—allopathic, autopathic, holistic, herbal, homeopathic, naturopathic ... and then decide on a course of action. Get copies of all reports and tests to add to your journal for future reference.

Be vigilant for certain health problems that are especially at risk of cropping up in a dog with cancer. A weekly home-care checkup is the best way to sidestep secondary illnesses and keep your dog healthy and strong during treatment.

Tumors

Check your dog's body for tumors regularly. This is very easy to do while you're giving him a massage. If you find any new lumps or bumps, inform your veterinarian.

Just two months after Bullet was diagnosed with lymphoma, Dr. Porzio examined a very small, pink, pimple-like growth near Bullet's ear. He said it had the appearance of a benign tumor and that we should watch it for any increase in size or change in appearance.

The tumor remained unchanged for a year but then suddenly grew to twice its original size. Dr. Hoskins removed it surgically as planned, using a short-acting anesthesia. One year later, another similar tumor developed at the base of Bullet's ear and was removed. The laboratory report on the excised tissue stated that these were both benign tumors.

Teeth

When a dog is in cancer treatment, dental hygiene is especially important. Chemotherapy can be destructive to teeth and gums. If your dog needs chemotherapy and has significant dental tartar and gingivitis, do not be surprised if your veterinarian wants to clean his teeth before treatment starts.

Chewing on bones is good for a dog's teeth. Even so, time will take its toll on tooth enamel and gums just as it does on humans, even though we brush twice a day. To avoid traumatic (not to mention expensive) dental cleanings and dental treatments, brush those pearly whites!

Brush your dog's teeth every other day. Be sure to use a toothpaste made for dogs or for human infants—one without any fluoride. A small amount of fluoride is good for our teeth, but it's actually a poison. People are capable of spitting out rather than swallowing, but dogs (and babies) are not. Toothbrushes for dogs are sold at pet supply stores; a child's toothbrush will work as well. There are toothpastes available for dogs, and you can also use toothpastes that are intended for a baby's teeth.

Brushing the front of your dog's teeth is sufficient. I know very few dogs good-natured enough to allow the inside surfaces of their teeth to be brushed.

If your dog isn't cooperative when you attempt to brush his teeth, introduce him to the process slowly. Settle him down, show him the brush, lift his lip, and make one quick stroke across his teeth. Give him a treat immediately. Do this one or more times a day, gradually upping the number of strokes each time. Most dogs become agreeable to the procedure quickly, especially if you find a flavored toothpaste that they like.

Eating frozen food may also be beneficial to a dog's tooth and gum health, although I've seen no research on this subject.

Elbows

Include a check for elbow sores in your routine whole-health checkup—the sores that dogs tend to develop from sleeping on hard surfaces. If you find such a sore, toss area rugs or mats over any hard surfaces on which your dog snoozes. If you suspect that the sores are infected (foul smelling, full of pus, swollen, or hot to the touch), inform your veterinarian right away.

I doused Bullet's elbow sores with hydrogen peroxide and applied an antibiotic ointment. I then either applied a wrap to prevent him from licking the medicine off, or I applied the medicine immediately before a walk or a feeding.

Nails, Pads, and Feet

During chemotherapy, a dog's nails may become brittle and crack easily. Because nails are constantly growing, they are subject to the ill effects of chemotherapy.

In August 2001, Bullet and I were out hiking, and I noticed that he was leaving bloody paw prints on the ground. I examined his feet to find that a nail had cracked off very close to its sheath. Once home, I pushed the open end of the nail into a bar of soap to stop the bleeding. Three more nails cracked off during the following month, but then the cracking ended. I increased the egg and tofu content of Bullet's diet to provide more protein, rubbed Musher's Secret into his nails and pads once a day, and kept his nails clipped short.

Since Bullet wasn't hiking and running as he did in his pre-cancer days, the fur between his toes grew long enough to cover the pads. This made for a slippery walking surface, evidenced by Bullet's difficulty in ascending the ramp to the car. Keeping the fur between his toes clipped short gave him better traction.

When a dog has difficulty walking for any reason, clip any fur growing between the toes. This is important after any leg surgery or amputation.

Coat

Because cancer cells divide more frequently than do healthy cells, chemotherapy agents are designed to attack cells that are in the process of dividing. As planned, the agents attack cancer cells, but healthy cells that happen to be in the process of cell division are also targeted.

People in chemotherapy often lose hair because protein-based cells such as hair and nails undergo cell division at a higher rate than do other cells. Dogs usually avoid this side effect, but don't forget to keep your dog's coat in good condition by bathing and grooming regularly.

It's common for dogs in chemotherapy to lose their whiskers. Bullet lost all of his whiskers three months after beginning treatment, and a few months after his last chemotherapy treatment, new whiskers appeared. They were somewhat scraggly, but Bullet didn't seem to mind.

Eighteen months after beginning treatment, Bullet lost his guard hair coat all at once. My herbalist recommended a supplement called silica and provided me with dried, ground nettles to sprinkle on his food. The fallout ended, but Bullet's guard hair coat never returned. To the end, he had a beautiful coat, but shorter, fluffier, and softer than the typical husky coat.

Stress and Pilling

Common sense tells us that stress is not good for a dog with cancer. Watch your dog for signs of stress. Every dog has a different set of stressors, so it's impossible to say just what to watch for. Any change in behavior could be an indication that your dog is feeling stressed.

When a dog is ill, pilling can become stressful, especially when there are many pills to be given over a long period of time. Putting a handful of medications and supplements down Bullet's throat three times daily would have been stressful for both of us.

▶ Food Plus Meds: If your dog is eating reliably, mix the pills that are not marked "on an empty stomach" with his food. If your dog is not eating reliably, possibly due to treatment side effects, this method will lead to the disposing of a great deal of uneaten food, along with medications.

▶ *PB & P:* Spread peanut butter or soy butter onto a bit of bread, press the pills into it, then fold it over to make a "peanut butter and pills" sandwich. If your dog is skilled at eating the bread and the spread, but spitting out the pills one by one, try another method.

▶ Pound Cake Plus: Mix pills and powders in a bowl with a bit of crumbled pound cake. This was our method of choice. Even when Bullet wasn't eating reliably, I could always persuade him to eat the "pound cake plus meds" combo.

An added advantage of using the "pound cake plus" method is that if your dog doesn't eat the offering, it's very easy to pick the pills out and try again later. Once pills have been mixed into a food bowl, they are difficult or impossible to retrieve.

▶ Mix Powder with Water: Use a needle-less syringe to mix the powder with filtered water. With a finger on the open end, shake to mix. Place the open end inside your dog's lips and slowly empty the contents into his mouth.

Many supplements are available in powder form rather than capsules. If this method works with your dog, buy the powder form when possible.

▶ Manual Pilling: There were times when I could not get Bullet to eat the pills no matter what. In these cases, I "pilled him" manually. Here's the method I used:
1. Stand next to your dog, facing the same direction.
2. With the hand nearest him, reach over his neck and under his chin. Insert your thumb and middle finger between his teeth, on either side of his lower jaw, just to the rear of his "fangs."
3. Gently but firmly pull down his lower jaw. Use the thumb of the other hand (holding pills) to lift the upper jaw; insert hand and pills.
4. Drop pills on his tongue as far back as you can, and remove all fingers.
5. Let his mouth close, but hold his head up a bit and stroke his neck until he swallows.

Wardrobe

The lymphatic system often plays a role in cancer. Often, enlarged lymph nodes are the first clue that a dog has cancer. So, it makes sense to avoid irritating a dog's lymph nodes. Dog collars press on the submandibular nodes. A harness is better than a collar, to avoid irritating the nodes and also to avoid tracheal collapse. But many harnesses cut in behind the front legs, applying pressure to the axillary nodes.

Look for a lymph node-friendly harness at www.Hug-A-Dog.com or www.RCPets.com, or choose one of the great harnesses offered by RuffWear, at www.RuffWear.com.

Vaccinations

The same vaccinations that protect our pets from a variety of ills may also put them in harm's way. Some cancers develop due to vaccines from repeated injections at the same site or from the adjuvants that are added into the vaccines. Beyond this understood cause and effect, research is under way to understand further what role vaccines play in the development of cancer. Dr. W. Jean Dodds, DVM, is an expert in this field and a leading investigator. Dr. Dodds was very kind to provide the following information specifically for this book:

"Vaccines are necessary and generally safe and effective, but can be harmful to dogs in selected situations. Natural immune surveillance mechanisms protect the body against cancer-causing agents. Vaccines may cause these protective mechanisms to fail.

Vaccination can overwhelm an immunocompromised dog. A dog with cancer is likely to be immunocompromised for two reasons: The presence of cancer cells can suppress immune function, and cancer treatment can also suppress immune function.

The cumulative effect of a lifetime of vaccinations may have dire consequences for a dog in later life."

So, titer test! If your dog does not have cancer, you must decide which vaccines you want him to have and which you want to decline. If there's a low incidence of a particular disease in your region, and if the treatment for it is effective and not painful, then the answer may be not to vaccinate. However, if there's a significant incidence of the disease in your region and there's no effective, safe, and economically viable treatment, then you might decide to vaccinate.

Ask Your Veterinarian
- ▶ What are the odds that your pet might contract the disease? What percentage of pets in your region had it in the past year?
- ▶ What's the efficacy of the vaccine? To what degree does it protect pets from the disease?
- ▶ Are there preventives other than vaccines? How effective are they?
- ▶ When a pet gets this disease, what is the treatment? Is it successful? Painful? Expensive?
- ▶ With treatment, what is the prognosis for dogs who contract this disease?

Weigh the risks of vaccinating against the risks of not vaccinating, research the incidence of the disease in your region and the efficacy of the preventive, and then make your best decision.

Whether or not to vaccinate a pet is up to the owner with the exception of the rabies vaccine, which is required by law in most states unless a waiver is accepted. See Vaccine Waiver in Appendix. Print the form and bring it to your veterinarian. Then send it to the state with the form that asks you to provide proof of vaccination.

A pet with cancer should not receive vaccinations.

Vaccine inserts give assurances that the vaccine can be safely given to a healthy pet. If your dog has cancer, he is not a healthy pet, and you can request a waiver from your state for any vaccines that are mandated, including the rabies vaccine. If you have an aggressive dog that would, under any circumstances, bite a person or a pet, do not waive the rabies vaccine. You may say that you have complete control over your dog and he will never ever bite anyone. But "stuff happens." Your dog could get loose and bite someone. When the person must undergo a series of injections that might or might not save his life, your excuses and apologies will fall short.

In *Natural Health for Dogs & Cats*, Dr. Richard Pitcairn warns, "Giving a vaccine to an animal with cancer is like pouring gasoline on a fire." Dr. Dodds reports that a dog's immune system may be compromised by vaccination for up to forty-five days and, after the rabies vaccine, longer.

The rabies vaccine is required by law in New York State. Bullet had a three-year rabies vaccine in October 1999, and when he was diagnosed with cancer in July 2000, I didn't think he would outlive the vaccine. In October 2002, the New York dog license renewal form arrived requesting proof of current rabies vaccination. My veterinarian filled out a waiver, which I enclosed with the renewal form and a check. The waiver was accepted without question, and Bullet's license to be a dog was renewed. He had no vaccines at all for his last four years and four months of life.

There is a serious risk involved in waiving a vaccine. An unvaccinated dog is at risk for contracting the rabies virus if bitten by an infected animal.

Aggressive dogs should always be given the Rabies vaccine. If an unvaccinated dog bites a person or another dog, even if the owner is absolutely sure that the dog has never been bitten or contacted by any creature that could have given him Rabies, he has to be tested for the virus. Testing requires examining the brain tissue after the dog is killed.

Preventives

Heartworm preventives and products that protect your dog from flea and tick bites may be problematic for a dog with cancer. Some veterinarians and some owners claim that these products should not be used on a dog with cancer; others claim that they are perfectly safe. There are varying opinions on this subject among veterinarians, and I have no strong belief in either position.

If you live in an area where heartworm disease, flea infestation, or tick bites are uncommon, you may decide to go without a preventive. Ask your veterinarian how many cases there have been in the past few years.

> *After Bullet's cancer diagnosis in the summer of 2000, I did not apply heartworm preventive or flea and tick repellent. In the summer of 2001, I feared I was pushing my luck and used Frontline® every three months and Interceptor® every month and a half. I considered this a compromise, since both products recommend more frequent applications. In the summer of 2002, I didn't use either. I was afraid to use them and afraid not to. I tried some "natural" preventives but they didn't work. I used the preventives every other year—and I prayed.*
>
> *When Bullet became ill in November 2002, I feared heartworm. He was coughing and gagging intermittently, and I cursed myself for not having used preventive. As it turned out, the cause of the coughing was not heartworm at all. It was heart failure.*

It is possible to avoid mainstream preventives, using natural products that may provide protection. Nosodes, for example, may protect a dog against a particular disease. Nosodes formulated for canine heartworm disease may protect a dog from the disease and can also be given as a remedy when a dog has heartworm disease. Nosodes are homeopathic remedies formulated from the disease itself, as are vaccines. Although they have been in use for many years, the efficacy of Nosodes is highly controversial. Brewer's yeast (mixed with a dog's food) and a variety of natural sprays can keep fleas and/or ticks at bay.

When vaccines are not given, periodic titer tests are extremely important. Consider titer testing twice a year for any disease against which your dog isn't being vaccinated.

Heartworm disease can be fatal but if detected early, it may be cured. Lyme and other tick-borne diseases often respond well to a course of antibiotics. If the diagnosis comes early and treatment is given right away, there is a good chance that the symptoms will vanish. Early detection results in the best prognosis. In some cases, the disease persists and can cause long-term lameness and/or neurologic symptoms.

Members of the Yahoo group "jstsayno2vaccs" use a homemade natural insect repellent with great success and no ill effects. "Aside from being effective against fleas, ticks, and mosquitoes," they say, "our horse and goat people swear by it to keep flies away from them as well!"

> ▸ Keep in the refrigerator—it will go musty/moldy if left at room temperature. Can usually be refrigerated for two to three weeks.
> ▸ Pour one quart of boiling water over the following ingredients:
> ▸ Rind of one grapefruit, rind of one lemon, rind of one lime, rind of one orange, and a handful of fresh rosemary and/or lavender (about a tablespoon of dried herbs).
> ▸ Let steep overnight. Strain through cheesecloth and put resulting liquid into mister/spray bottle. Lightly mist yourself and the dogs before outdoor jaunts. Use this repellent several times per day if necessary.

First-Aid Kit For a Dog With Cancer

Our four-legged family members seem to find a way to get into the most unexpected predicaments, and they manage to almost always do it late at night or on a weekend. It's a good idea for any pet owner to have a doggie first aid kit handy. Those who have a dog with cancer can add the following items to the kit:

Glutamine and Colostrum

Dogs in chemotherapy often have gastrointestinal side effects from their treatments. The side effects generally show up about five days after a treatment, when the damaged cells from the lining of the small intestine are being expelled. Glutamine will help the lining heal. If there is blood in the stool or diarrhea, also give colostrum.

Pepcid® AC

If the treatment has damaged the stomach lining or the first section of the small intestine, an ulcer may be forming. If your dog won't eat, try giving Pepcid® AC and then offer food about twenty minutes later.

Elderberry Syrup

If you suspect that your dog is nauseous, this will help to make him feel better. It works on people too!

Pepto-Bismol® Chewable Wafers for Diarrhea

Flagyl

Good for mucousy stools. This is a prescription drug that is an antibiotic with anti-inflammatory effects.

Pain Medication

Ask your veterinarian to make a recommendation. This is a must for any dog that is in palliative care.

Rescue® Remedy

A homeopathic Bach flower essence remedy, for stress.

Gurney

If you have a large dog, make or buy a gurney-type device or a cart on wheels that will enable you to transport him to help if he's unable to walk.

Where Are You Going?

In my experience and in compliance with Murphy's Law, pets become ill most often late on Saturday, on a Sunday, or late at night on a weekday. Locate a twenty-four-hour veterinary clinic nearby. Program the clinic's phone number into your cell phone and write (or print) directions to keep in your car or wallet. Take a test drive to be sure that you will be able to find the clinic quickly if necessary.

If there is no emergency clinic near you, ask your veterinarian to give you an emergency phone number, so you can contact him during the night if necessary.

If you travel, share this information with the person who cares for your dog while you are away. If you want to empower the sitter to make emergency decisions about your dog's care in your absence, let your clinic know.

When you travel with your dog, do a little research before leaving home to locate the nearest veterinary clinic and, if possible, the nearest veterinary oncologist and/or twenty-four-hour clinic. Also bring your dog's medical records along (in your journal) to help an unfamiliar veterinarian become familiar with your dog's medical history quickly.

13

From Warrior to Angel

T he special bond that you have with your dog grows stronger over time and deepens when your dog requires special attention. You invest a great deal of time, effort, and emotional and physical energy into helping your dog fight cancer.

Hope and pray that treatment will be a complete success, even though you know that in most cases cancer is not cured. Hope more realistically that treatment will prolong, delay, or postpone the inevitable.

When a dog is diagnosed with cancer, we don't know how this dog will respond to treatment. We don't know if this dog will get a miracle and survive cancer-free for the rest of his life, or if he will not tolerate treatment and die before the prognosis predicts. All we can do is *try*. We toss the dice and hope for a miracle.

From Comet's Mom

I hope I made the right decision as I do not want to lose him yet…I know I am just prolonging the inevitable, but he is so young, and I love him dearly. I am grasping at every little bit of hope there is.

Making the decision to end treatment and begin pawspice (palliative or hospice) care may be the hardest thing you'll ever have to do. You will say, "The battle against cancer is over, and now I will provide pawspice care and maintain a good quality of life for my beloved dog, without pain or suffering, for as long as possible."

Now your dog is no longer a warrior and you are no longer fighting an unbeatable foe, tilting against windmills like Don Quixote. Now it's all about quality of life and treasuring every moment of time you have left together.

When your dog enters pawspice (palliative care), you will stop all treatments, therapies, and home-care modalities that may result in adverse results. Give only the treatments or remedies that might help him survive longer without risking side effects. Do what you can to delay the decline but don't use anything that might make him sick.

Continue exercise, supplements, and a healthy diet. Provide all of the things that your dog loves. Take lots of photographs and videos—they will be very valuable when pawspice care ends.

The decision to give up the fight may invoke feelings of helplessness, guilt, and anticipatory grief. Strive not to allow any of these feelings to distract you from the task of making every moment a good one. There will be time for sadness later.

While your dog is still with you, celebrate that fact. Don't bury your head in the blankets and cry. Get up and play with your dog! Sometime soon you will not be able to do that anymore.

You have given your dog a wonderful life. When it is time to give up the fight, you will do everything you can to ensure that your dog has a good end-of-life experience and eventually a good death.

When Pawspice Begins

When Treatment Ends and Palliative Care Begins

▶ When treatment is not effective and there are no other treatment options with any promise of success.

▶ When your dog is suffering "too much" from the effects of the disease or of the treatment. This is a judgment call that only you can make. You are the one who can evaluate your dog's quality of life, his level of suffering, and his ability to continue the battle.

▶ When you determine that it's time to stop fighting because you, your family, or your dog can no longer keep up the fight.

▶ Your veterinarian may be the first to suggest that it's time for pawspice to begin. For help making the decision, ask the most compassionate member of your team.

Beginning pawspice care doesn't mean you are going to give up and simply allow your dog to die. Pawspice care can go on for quite a long time, depending on the situation. There is a lot to be done during this last part of your dog's life.

Words Matter

During this inevitable phase of pet care, a small word can have a profound emotional effect. Some terms may make you flinch—pay attention and be kind to yourself. When you speak, write or think about this event, use gentle words that will honor your pet and also give you solace.

Say "The beginning of pawspice or of palliative care."
When no more treatment will be given, for whatever reason, this is the beginning of pawspice care. Instead of calling this the end of treatment or a failure, let's call it the beginning of something.

At the end of pawspice, say "Helped my dog go to the Rainbow Bridge."
This describes the final gift we are empowered to give our pets, to release them from pain. "Put him to sleep" misrepresents what has happened. Not to mention the fear that it can instill in a child. Hearing this euphemism used about the end of a dog's life, and then about the child's bedtime can be confusing.

"Put him down" is impersonal and devaluing. "Euthanasia" is clinical and cold.

Say "Passed," or "Went to Rainbow Bridge."
The Rainbow Bridge is a fabled place that helps us through pet loss and grief. It is not religious and if accepted as a fable, we can think of it as a comforting way to think of the loss. Rainbow Bridge comes from a beautiful poem attributed to Paul C. Daum. For a lovely video rendition of the poem, go to www.indigo.org/rainbowbridge_ver2.html.

"Died" is harsh.
"Passed on" is evasive.
"Transitioned." Well, okay … if you insist.

Decide and Forget

It's important to make preparations, if you haven't already done so. Plan for the end before the end. Make your plans when the end is not yet near. Making decisions about your pet's end of life is not a pleasant task, but having your plans set will alleviate anxiety later. Make these decisions now, with a clear mind.

When the end does come, you will not have to panic about what is going to happen. You will be able to give your dog a sweet, calm last day with no drama or last-minute decisions. Make these decisions and then forget about them. Get back to providing your dog with a beautiful, happy, loving last phase of life.

Emergency or Planned Euthanasia

Find out if your veterinarian is available at night or on weekends. If not, try to find a twenty-four-hour clinic near you. If your dog is in pain on a Saturday or Sunday, or in the middle of the night, you will need to know where you can take him for help.

Pain Management

Pain is the number one factor in QoL. When pawspice begins, start watching for signs of pain, including decreases in appetite, activity, social interaction, and stamina.

Have pain medicine on hand. Dogs can be given nonsteroidal anti-inflammatory drugs (NSAIDs). There are many pharmaceuticals that can help as well. Discuss with your veterinarian which type of pain medication makes sense for you to have for your dog.

The "Pain Management Guidelines for Dogs and Cats," recently released by the AAHA/AAFP Pain Management Task Force, will help your veterinarian recommend the best medications to control or manage your dog's pain. Task Force co-chair Dr. Susan Downing, states, "Old age is not a disease. Many of the behaviors we previously attributed to aging are actually driven by pain."

Final Resting Place

Will your dog be cremated? Find a crematory and write down the phone number, hours, pick-up services, and days of operation. You can choose private cremation, where your dog will be cremated alone and the cremains that you receive will be only his. Or you can choose group cremation. The cost difference is significant. Ask when your dog's cremains would be returned to you and in what type of container or urn.

If you prefer a burial, decide where. A pet cemetery? Make the arrangements now. At home? The winter ground is hard in some parts of the country, so if you're planning an at home burial, prepare a plot in advance and have a casket, or a box of the correct size, ready.

Use the Quality of Life Scale

While a dog is in pawspice, owners are fearful that they will not know when it is time for euthanasia. Many fear that they will miss the signs and that their dog will suffer. Dr. Alice Villalobos developed a very useful tool called the HHHHHMM Quality of Life Scale. (See Appendix.)

Print it out. Print several copies. Whenever there is a change in your dog's condition, fill it out again. Adding up your responses will help you decide whether or not your dog's QoL is high enough to continue providing pawspice care.

There are many factors to consider, including his ability to do the things he loves most, his mobility, and his ability to eat and drink, urinate, and defecate.

The most important factor to consider is your dog's degree of pain and suffering. Uncontrollable pain and suffering are clear signs that it is time for pawspice to end; that your warrior is ready to become an angel.

> *Dr. Porzio and I discussed various rescue therapies used for dogs relapsing from a remission. We agreed that, if and when Bullet came out of remission, we would call on our board-certified veterinary oncologist consultant, Dr. Dave Ruslander, for guidance.*
>
> *We also discussed what would happen "at the end." We agreed on a course of action. The conversation gave me a comforting sense of preparedness and alleviated my anxieties.*
>
> *When I got home, I called the pet crematorium in my area, Hartsdale Pet Cemetery & Crematory. I asked about their hours and what I should do if their services were needed, for example, on a Sunday night. I asked about the cremation procedure and the prices.*
>
> *With the plan of action settled, I put the printed information on my bulletin board, and it stayed there for four and a half years, until I needed it.*

Make these decisions and then put them aside. During Pawspice, keep the focus on making the last days or weeks happy ones. Do your best to stay strong for your dog now. Do not grieve during this time. There will be time to grieve later.

When Pawspice Ends

People with pets in pawspice care invariably ask me, *"Will I know?"* My response is always, *"You will know!"* I've assured hundreds of people, and I can always hear that they are not convinced. They are afraid that they will not make the decision at the right time. Yet, each and every one told me later that I was right—they *did* know.

Trust your connection with and your knowledge of your dog. Trust the bond. We have the ability and the responsibility to decide when our pets' lives will end. Medical team members and support group members may help by suggesting that the time is near or that the time is now. Their advice is invaluable, but we must ultimately make this decision on our own. Sometime later, we will know that we did right by our friend.

> *We'd all like our pets to die at home, peacefully, in our arms, with no pain. Once in a while, the universe is kind and grants us this wish. It did for Bullet, and I am very grateful for that.*
>
> *When Bullet went to the Rainbow Bridge on November 20, 2004, I began to revive him but stopped. It occurred to me later that he had a good death and if I had revived him, the next one might not be so good. I knew that it wouldn't have been a long revival in any case.*

Often, pawspice ends with euthanasia. Many veterinarians offer at home euthanasia. The family and dog are relaxed in their own space, with loved ones. If this is your preference, call the clinic to find out if at home euthanasia is available, when an appointment would have to be scheduled, and the fee.

If euthanasia is at the clinic, some clinics have a special room for the procedure, with candles and a CD player so that families can bring special music. Staff members are respectful and do not interrupt, or they attend, to offer the family support. If the veterinarians at your clinic don't provide an atmosphere of respect and compassion for euthanasia, please educate them.

Even though we know that euthanasia is the right thing to do, it is hard. It is almost impossible. But we do it anyhow, out of love. Helping a suffering dog get to the Rainbow Bridge is the most important gift we can give. It is the ultimate sacrifice because, at this point, their suffering ends and ours begins.

In some ways, the loss of a pet is like any loss. Grief is grief. In some ways, this loss is unlike any other. It is different because our pets do not grow up and move away. They are with us forever. It is different because we have the ability and the *responsibility* to make end-of-life decisions for them.

Having the right to make these choices is an *ability* because we are enabled and empowered to make choices that will spare our friends pain and suffering when there is no hope of recovery.

Having this right is also a *responsibility*. It is our *responsibility* to make use of our ability, our power, our right, to make this momentous decision on behalf of our pet. Unfortunately, as a consequence of making the decision, we are left feeling *responsible* for having ended the dog's life. We may second-guess ourselves. We may question our wisdom and decide, in grief and self-loathing, that we made a horrible mistake. What an unbearably heavy weight to carry.

At the moment that a dog's pain and suffering ends, the owner's begins. It is a choice, an ability, and a responsibility, to take on hardship so that our dogs don't have to. It's a sacrifice. It's a gift.

After the Loss

Almost all owners experience a deep sense of guilt after the loss of a pet. The responsibility to choose a time rests on our shoulders, and it is huge. A sense of urgency is involved in making this decision at exactly the right moment—not too early and not too late. Every day, I speak to owners who are stressed about their ability to decide.

"Too early" means that we deprived our dog of more time and

ourselves of more time in his company. An owner may suspect or imagine that he ended his dog's life too early, but there is absolutely no way to know this for sure. The hope is that euthanasia was performed at just the right time and that otherwise the dog would have suffered. I believe our special connection to our dog informs us when this will happen if we do not act.

"Too late" is more difficult. It means that the dog suffered, and anyone who takes this responsibility to heart does his or her level best not to wait until the pain has set in. Unfortunately, as you may know from experience, this is not always possible. If your dog experiences pain before you are able to help him to the Rainbow Bridge, remember that the duration of their pain was negligible in comparison to the long, wonderful life that your dog had with you.

In recent years, the position that pets fill in their owners' lives has been upgraded. Some of us acknowledge and value our pets as four-legged family members. Others consider the family dog or cat, rabbit, gerbil, or ferret to be no more meaningful—and sometimes less valuable—than a piece of furniture. The latter group is not terribly concerned about pet loss, and the following does not apply to them.

For the bonded owner, a loss is followed by excruciating grief. Very often, that grief is tinged with guilt—sometimes terrible guilt. This grief is part of pet loss in particular because we are so completely responsible for making that final decisions for our pets.

We think, "*If I had made different choices, my dog would still be here.*" In every end-of-life situation, there are things that could have been done differently. We make the best decisions we can. And then, we must believe that our decisions were the best ones available.

Measuring Grief

You probably have friends and family who do not have pets, or who are not especially bonded with their pets. They do not understand. They complain, "*That's enough, it's time to move on!*" They may say, "*Get over it, he was only a dog!*" These comments may be meant to help, but they are insulting and infuriating. If you feel compelled to voice objections and defend yourself—don't! Doing so will only lead to further frustration and will not change their point of view.

I read many pet loss books when Bullet went to the Bridge. I had to laugh when I found a chapter in one of the books titled "Overly Bonded Owners." The author of that book would likely include you and me in that group, but that is a group of which I am proud to be a member.

Avoid speaking about your loss to those who do not understand. If you are surrounded by people who don't understand, join an online support group. You are certainly not alone and there is nothing wrong about your bond with your dog, or your need to grieve.

Find Support

Do not minimize the effect that your loss has on you emotionally and on all aspects of your life. If you cannot cope with the sadness, please find help.

Attend a pet loss support group. Many shelters and animal hospitals offer them. Your veterinarian may be able to refer you to one. Often, the group leader is a mental health professional who you can trust to step in if more help is needed. The leader may counsel you privately as well, if you feel this would help.

There are many pet loss support groups online.

My friend Connie lives in a very rural area where there are no pet loss support groups, and she does not use a computer. Connie appealed to a local human hospice and was accepted with open arms to share her grief in their support group.

If you're more comfortable one-on-one, find a private therapist with experience in bereavement or grief counseling.

Light Memorial Candles

When Bullet passed, I lit a seven-day candle that gave me great solace and comfort. I placed the glass-enclosed pillar candle near the spot where Bullet spent his last days. The flickering flame had a profound effect on me. It symbolized him, his spirit, his presence, and his absence. After seven days, when the flame was about to flicker out, I rushed out to the store in a panic to buy a new one. I just needed to see the flame dancing there for another week.

* If you light candles in memory of your pet, be sure to position them safely so that there is no danger of starting a fire.

Display Photographs and Videos

Create an album for your dog. Use photographs and any video clips you have, to create a slide show on your computer. You can e-mail your slide show to friends and family, or copy it onto a CD or DVD and mail copies out, in tribute to your sweet dog.

While handling images and remembering the moments they were taken, allow your mind to wander back to the good, happy times captured in each image.

Make a project of it. Select the most special photos of your dog. Frame and hang them on the walls of your home.

Hold a Memorial Service

Gather together the people who knew and loved your dog, for the purpose of paying tribute. Don't forget to invite your veterinarian and clinic staff. They are family too! There's no "right" time.

I had a memorial service for Bullet a month after he went to the Bridge. Twenty people came, and we formed a circle around an easel holding a big photograph of Bullet, with his urn beside it. I read a passage I had prepared. Bullet's godfather (and my Yoga teacher), Ru Schwager chanted a prayer. Each person around the circle told a story about Bullet. Finally, we all walked a half-mile trail called Peaceful Path, a trail that Bullet and I had traveled together thousands of times.

Expression is the Opposite of Depression

You kept a journal during your dog's illness. Now keep one during the days and weeks after your loss. Write your thoughts and feelings down to document your pet loss journey. Later, reading this journal, you will revisit the wonderful feeling of your dog having just recently been in your arms.

Cling to moments just after the loss, when your dog is still "in the air." It is painful that he isn't there, but at least his presence will linger in his favorite places, in your head and in your heart.

As time passes, his presence will not be as strong. You will grieve and then you will begin to heal from the painful loss. As this happens, your dog's presence will become less strong. And then, I predict, you will wish you could make it come back.

Read "So Easy to Love, So Hard to Lose"

My pet loss book may help you through pawspice and the loss. I very carefully sequenced the reading and the journaling to inform you, lead you and help you through the journey step by step. Each person grieves differently, but I think you will find that you can relate to the progression of thoughts and feelings discussed in the book.

Reading the text pages will help you understand, normalize, and validate your experience. Writing answers on the project pages will help you bring forward the thoughts and feelings that will help you walk strongly through the pet loss experience and create a tribute to your dog.

Bullet's Story

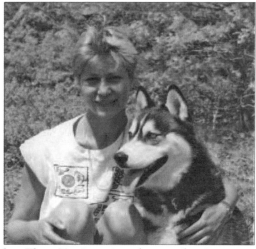

On September 19, 1992, I was toying with the idea of sharing my home with a dog in addition to my three cats, KC, Bumi, and TipToe. I wandered into my local SPCA, where I had adopted TipToe a year earlier, but intended only to hand out biscuits to the pups.

My friend Kevin and I handed out the treats to many of the dogs, and we took a few for walks in the shelter parking lot. Then Kevin pointed out a dog in a large kennel that was housing several medium-to-large dogs. The ID tag hanging on the cage indicated that this was Max, an eighteen-month-old neutered male Siberian husky. Max was sitting quietly amid the chaos generated by the other dogs, all barking wildly and vying for position to receive biscuits.

Max had the most beautiful ears and eyes I'd ever seen. He was strikingly black and white with a handsome star-shaped design on his chest. I looked at Max and he looked at me. It was unnerving, being studied with such intensity by two icy blue eyes in a canine head. Love at first sight? Maybe so—in any case, I knew then and there that this dog was going home with me.

According to the shelter manager, Max had been relinquished by his owner the previous day. The owner complained that Max was an escape artist and a "runner." He had to retrieve Max from the local police department's animal control unit—for a fee—one time too many.

I've since learned, by reading about the breed and by chasing Bullet down so many times, that it is redundant to say a dog is a Siberian husky and that he is a runner. In fact, I had an opportunity to witness the Siberian penchant for escape on our very first day. I had Max taken from his kennel, and I walked him in the parking lot. I left Kevin holding the leash, and I went into the office to pay the suggested $40 donation. When I came out a few minutes later, I found Kevin still holding the leash … only now the leash was dangling to the ground with no dog attached to it. When Kevin noticed my expression, he said, "Oh, *you're taking that dog?*"

A shelter worker, Kevin, and I all set out to chase Max down. He was having great fun watching the three of us over his shoulder as he ran, and eluding all of our attempts at capture. Finally, exasperated, I stopped running, clapped my hands and yelled *"MAAAAX!"* To everyone's amazement, Max ran right to me from behind a nearby house and rolled over on his back at my feet—an event that would never ever happen again.

Soon thereafter, Max became Bullet (as in faster than a speeding bullet) because of his great love of running. His friends called him "Bully" because of his great love of growling.

During our first six months together, Bullet was expelled from three boarding kennels, and two dog trainers proclaimed him untrainable. One went so far as to recommend that I return him to the shelter. Alas, it was too late. I suspect it was too late from the moment that I put him in my car at the SPCA.

Bullet destroyed everything that was not nailed down, and a few things that were. He loved nothing more than to chew on (but never bite) a human hand or arm. Periodically, I had to go into another room and close the door to give myself a "time out" from Bullet. I was exhausted from yelling "NO!" over and over. I came across the movie *Turner and Hooch* and howled with laughter. I related completely to Turner's frustration and exasperation (played by Tom Hanks).

As a strong, healthy youth, Bullet was a big-time puller on leash. If only I had a nickel for every time a passerby said, *"Who's walking whom?"* I didn't weigh much more than Bullet, and he was quite capable of pulling me right off my feet—especially if a squirrel, rabbit, or cat happened by to provide incentive.

When Bullet encountered unfamiliar dogs, he became extremely agitated, and I was never entirely sure whether he intended to play or fight. I would drag him off-trail, grab onto a tree, and just hang onto it until the dog passed by. But he loved all people and was always happy to allow anyone and everyone to pet him and admire him.

True to the breed, Bullet continued to run away whenever possible. He could chew through a nylon or leather leash so quickly and surreptitiously that he would be on the run with a healthy head start by the time I'd realize that he wasn't attached anymore. He even managed to get away from one of his trainers—it was the one who later suggested that I return him to the shelter.

I knew there was nothing wrong with this dog that a lot of tender love (and a lot of tough love) couldn't fix. I read dog-training books and books about the Siberian husky personality. I read in one book that if you want a master-slave relationship with your dog, do not get a Siberian.

At the start of the Westminster Kennel Club Dog Show, when Roger A. Caras was the announcer, he provided a commentary about each breed. He always said that the Siberian husky is an intelligent breed and highly trainable, but only if the trainer is more intelligent than the dog. I wondered if I would be able to train Bullet. I was prepared to take the challenge and find out who was more intelligent.

Bullet was a ridiculously high-maintenance dog. In time, he became a very opinionated but manageable dog. After some months, Bullet became more manageable. After a few years of training (which a friend used to call "Laurie's Boot Camp"), Bullet and I found a place of mutual respect with me as the alpha, albeit by a slim margin. The older he got, the better he got, and later, in his geriatric years, he was darn near perfect.

Bullet mastered the basic obedience commands, such as sit, down, stay, paw, other paw, jump, speak, and kiss (our favorite). But he never did learn to "Come" off lead. I decided that it must be a hearing problem. Bullet's hearing was just fine with a leash attached or in the house, but he reliably went stone-cold deaf the moment the leash was clicked off from the collar. From talking to other frustrated and bemused Siberian owners, I decided this hearing problem is genetic and breed related.

At first, Bullet slept in my finished basement at night. I had planned to introduce him to the cats gradually before allowing him free run of the house. I went downstairs each morning to find the floor littered with remnants of books, note pads, computer disks, pencils, and anything else within his reach. My friend Joe, who had lived with malamutes, convinced me that because Bullet was a Northern-breed dog, he should sleep outdoors. In light of the wreckage, this sounded to me like a great idea.

Bullet slept in the great outdoors, with his collar hooked onto an overhead run between two trees fifty feet apart. He had a doghouse full of hay, but turned up his nose at creature comforts. Bullet always slept under the stars, on a pile of hay outside of his doghouse, at the foot of an ash tree. In inclement weather, I brought him indoors to sleep, for his safety and comfort and for my peace of mind.

Bullet needed a water bowl in his outdoor home. During the winter, a dog's tongue can tear on frozen-over water. I had an electrical outlet installed next to the doghouse and plugged in a heated water bowl. To make further use of the outlet, I plugged in a baby monitor and placed it in the doghouse. I hung the monitor's receiver component beside my bed. More often than I care to remember, I was awakened in the wee hours by frantic barking through the monitor. Then came the de-skunking bath in the front yard in the middle of the night, and a car ride in search of a dumpster while holding a multi-wrapped skunk carcass out of the window, as far as possible from my nose.

I had a five-foot high chain link fence installed in the woods behind my house. The resulting dog pen measured fifty feet by fifty feet—larger than the footprint of my house. Furnished with a doghouse, lounge chair, and flat-roofed eating shed, this pen gave Bullet freedom from the overhead run, put a stop to the skunk carnage, and became "Bully's World."

Bullet taught me how to train an "untrainable" dog. He taught me to understand dog-speak and to communicate with him in a way that he could understand. But he taught me much more than that. Bullet inspired me to learn to knit so that I could make sweaters, vests, and scarves from his fur. Dog fur becomes fuzzy when knitted, looking very much like mohair, and the final product is so warm that I was unable to wear my Bully sweaters indoors. I turned sweaters into vests by removing the sleeves and, so as not to waste any precious fur, I turned the detached sleeves into slipper-socks.

Bullet also taught me to mush. On winter weekends, we went on dog sledding trips in Lake Placid, NY. There, he added a few new commands to his repertoire: hike (start running), gee (turn right), haw (turn left), straight on, and whoa. On these weekend trips, usually with my friend Kevin, I rented a cabin and a sled and three huskies from the owner of a professional dog sledding team. What a rush! Seeing Bullet take to sledding like a duck to water gave me new respect for who he was and for the natural order of things.

Bullet acquired a new nickname when my friend Tracy Basile visited an American Indian reservation. On her return, she was inspired to assign new names to our dogs. Her dogs, Kai (lionhearted deer dog, friend of the coyotes) and Toshi (frog dancer, water prancer) were Bullet's best furry friends for many years. During a solemn naming ceremony, we appropriately dubbed my ornery little boy "Bullet Growly Bear."

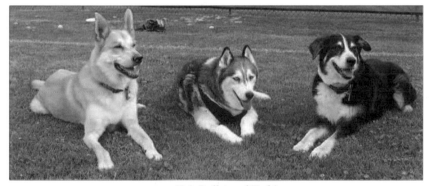

Kai, Bullet and Toshi

Tracy and I hired a trainer to work with our three big boys once a week, teaching them (and us) agility as well as reinforcing and refining their basic obedience. The trainer, Inez, added the commands jump, tunnel, and hoop to Bullet's vocabulary.

When Bullet was seven, he had arthroscopic surgery on both shoulders to remove a bone chip and debris from his shoulder joints. This marked the end of Bullet's sledding days and squashed any fantasies I had of participating in the Iditarod.

By then, two of my cats had died at ripe old ages. The third, TipToe, moved next door to spend a couple of weeks with my friend and neighbor, Margaret Kenny. I wanted Bullet to recuperate from his surgery indoors, and I wanted to remove the risk of re-injury due to chasing TipToe around the house. Bullet became a house dog, and he made this transition without complaint.

TipToe and Margaret fell in love. TipToe stayed next door, and the couple of weeks turned into eight years, until June 2006, when Margaret passed away at ninety-one years old. By that time, Bullet was no longer with me. TipToe moved back into my house and survived until December 23, 2010. When she was just over 19 years old, TipToe's kidneys failed.

Bullet's recovery from his shoulder surgery was difficult. My unruly, rebellious, and fiercely independent dog had become dependent. Bullet did regain his strength and his air of independence, but lost a little bit of his craziness. He was finally, at seven years old, starting to become a mature dog.

Bullet loved to lie under the table during my weekly bridge games, waiting for someone to sneak him a pizza crust under the table. He greeted visitors at the door and was always happy to wrestle with anyone willing to endure his mock-vicious growls and attacks. I often thought Bullet would be a perfect dog star for movies needing a dog who could look and sound vicious, but actually be harmless and safe to have on the movie set.

In May 2000, I felt enlarged nodes on Bullet, just where a doctor would feel your neck if you complained of a sore throat. Initially, our veterinarian suspected allergies and prescribed antihistamines. When the nodes remained large despite medication, I brought Bullet back for another exam. At this exam, the nodes were larger, and other nodes had become enlarged as well. Now the diagnosis of cancer became a more obvious possibility.

Bullet's lifelong primary care veterinarian, Dr. Bruce Hoskins, DVM, at Croton Animal Hospital in Croton-on-Hudson, NY, attempted a needle biopsy of a lymph node in order to rule out lymphoma. Because the fluid that he extracted did not contain any lymph fluid, the result was not helpful. So I agreed to a surgical biopsy.

Dr. Hoskins took the surgical biopsy tissue sample from an enlarged lymph node—the popliteal node, behind Bullet's knee. The node all but disintegrated during the procedure, Dr. Hoskins said, so he removed the node entirely.

The next evening, on July 17, 2000, Dr. Hoskins called to say, that the biopsy report was positive for lymphoma. I knew that this could not be true. There must be a mistake! Aside from the swollen glands in his neck, Bullet was a strong, healthy dog. Surely, the laboratory got their blood samples mixed up or had misinterpreted the results. I was assured that there is no mistake.

I was dumfounded. I was shocked. I had a lump in my throat and a knot in my stomach. I stayed up all night, intermittently hugging Bullet, crying, researching canine lymphoma online, and contacting anyone and everyone I knew in veterinary medicine or cancer research for advice. Without treatment, a dog with lymphoma will only survive a few weeks. It was very hard for me to grasp that my seemingly healthy dog could be so close to death.

Dr. Hoskins provided the names and telephone numbers of a couple of local veterinary oncologists, plus one local veterinarian who was not board-certified in oncology but provided cancer treatment to dogs and cats. This was Dr. Paolo Porzio. Dr. Porzio was at an animal hospital just half an hour away. I called the clinic, and Dr. Porzio agreed to start Bullet on chemotherapy the very next day.

The most important thing was to begin Bullet's treatment as soon as possible. I chose Dr. Porzio based on location and availability, despite the fact that he was not board-certified in oncology. I was under the impression that it would be better to have a veterinary oncologist provide chemotherapy. I thought we would begin treatment, and then I would take the time to research my options and find a specialist to continue the treatments.

During our first visit, however, I knew that Dr. Porzio was the right veterinarian to provide Bullet's long-term treatment. He spoke clearly, explained everything to me in an unrushed manner, and took his time answering all of my many questions thoroughly. Dr. Porzio had completed a residency in internal medicine in Saskatchewan. There was no staff oncologist at the school at the time, so the class had to learn to provide cancer treatment for the local dogs. The location appealed to me because not all veterinarians are enamored of the exuberance and obstinate nature of the Siberian husky. In Saskatchewan, Dr. Porzio would have become familiar with the many idiosyncrasies and antics of the breed.

Dr. Porzio was attentive to Bullet during our consultation and spoke to him in a gentle and affectionate manner. His bedside manner was perfect. Even the clinic was situated well for our needs. It was on the ground floor, and the storefront was a huge plate-glass window. Before entering, I could see if there were any dogs in the waiting room—a big plus, since Bullet didn't always take kindly to new dogs. It was a relief to know that there would never be a ruckus in the waiting room or a struggle to keep Bullet from tugging on the leash toward another dog in the waiting room.

Dr. Porzio treated canine lymphoma with a single-agent chemotherapy protocol using one drug repeatedly—doxorubicin. It was a stroke of luck for me and for Bullet that I was, at that time, editor-in-chief of a medical newsmagazine from Tufts University School of Veterinary Medicine called *Catnip*. I consulted Dr. David Ruslander, who was then at Tufts Vet School. Dr. Ruslander recommended that instead, we treat Bullet with a protocol called VELCAP-L. It was a more complex protocol, he said, but was showing a higher success rate.

Dr. Porzio agreed to administer the VELCAP-L protocol to Bullet under Dr. Ruslander's guidance. Dr. Ruslander provided excellent guidance during this protocol, and continued to contribute to Bullet's well-being and survival for years afterward.

Once I had a medical treatment plan in place, I wanted to know, *"What else can I do?"* I made an appointment with a local holistic vet, who spoke

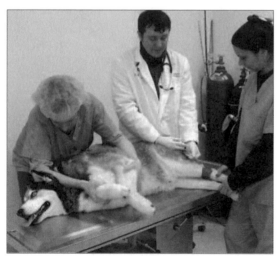

to me of the many dogs who survived cancer under his care. He showed me before and after pictures, and he attributed their survival to the treatment that he had provided. Dr. Marty Goldstein gave me my first lesson in holistic cancer support for dogs.

I was off and running, and ready to settle in for what I hoped would be a long haul. The initial panic and fear had subsided, and I prepared to fine-tune Bullet's treatment and home care and to spend as much time as possible treasuring every single moment of borrowed time with my beautiful boy.

Throughout Bullet's seventy-five-week chemotherapy protocol, I saw him as a cancer dog. My thoughts about him were tinged by the inevitability that at some time—perhaps today or perhaps a year from today—his remission would lapse; he would have chemotherapy side effects; he would slip into cancer cachexia.

When someone we love is diagnosed with a terminal illness, our feelings for that person are altered. That "someone" may be a cat or a dog just as easily as a human—it can be any living creature that has won our love. I never took Bullet for granted, but after his diagnosis, my constant vigilance of and concern about his physical health and his quality of life intensified. I didn't think it was possible, but my connection to him became even stronger.

When I adopted Bullet at 18 months old, my friend Diane said that each time Bullet would have an illness or injury in the future, our bond would deepen.

From July 2000 forward, during Bullet's cancer journey, Diane's words resonated. Before the diagnosis, when Bullet was nine years old, I would not have believed our bond could become stronger. But it did become ever stronger, deeper, and more infinite.

Bullet began the VELCAP-L chemotherapy protocol July 18, 2000, and completed it in March 2002. He was nine and a half years old going into chemotherapy, and eleven coming out. I was offended the first time Dr. Hoskins referred to Bully as a "geriatric dog." How dare he! Ironically, after I got used to the concept, I often referred to Bullet as a geriatric dog with great pride.

During Bullet's long protocol, he was worn down. During the six months that followed his last treatment, Bullet's posture, coat quality, eating habits, and energy level—even his facial expressions—changed for the better. Once again he was strong, full of energy, playful, and happy.

Without chemotherapy, Bullet would certainly have had no chance of survival longer than the typical four-to-six-week period predicted for dogs with untreated lymphoma. It may be that Bullet's survival so far beyond his prognosis was due simply to his hardy constitution and his extremely stubborn personality.

As Bullet regained his willful, playful husky personality, we fell back into our old routine of arguing over which trail to hike, which toy to toss around, when to get into or out of the car, and other very important decisions. He was again able to climb Anthony's Nose, part of the Bear Mountain range, and spend long weekends with his furry friends running on the beach in Cape Cod.

Bullet was well traveled. I never put him on a plane, but he was a wonderful road trip companion. His self-proclaimed place in my car was sitting with body in the back and chest and paws on the center console. If there were other dogs in the car, they best not attempt to claim this "shotgun" seat of honor. Any attempt to supplant him was met with a demonstration of how he obtained his nickname, "Bullet Growly Bear."

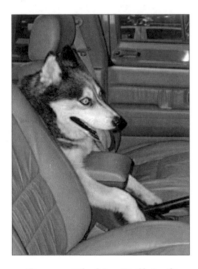 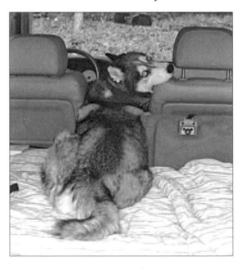

Once settled in, Bullet often rested his head in the crook of my right arm while I was driving. It was perfectly positioned, that head, so I could easily lean over to kiss it at red lights. When Bully became drowsy on a long trip, the full weight of that handsome two-ton head would make my right arm ache and fall asleep.

Apart from our many trips to Cape Cod, our journeys included Lake Placid for sledding when Bullet was young; Washington, DC to visit my cousins; and Big Indian, NY, for long weekends of snowshoeing in the winter and hiking in the summer. We also took trips to Killington, VT; Paoli, PA; Oneonta, NY; Boston, MA; and the Delaware Water Gap, where Bullet stood his ground at our campsite and ferociously scared off a brown bear (while I was frantically dragging him into the car). Bullet was a great tent camper. He was always a well-behaved guest at hotels, inns, and in friends' homes. One of his favorite things was taking an elevator ride down to the lobby of a hotel and being surrounded by children wanting to hug and pet him when the doors opened. I may be anthropomorphizing, but he seemed to me to be disappointed when the doors opened and no one was there to hug him.

After years of remission, I was able to look at Bullet without thoughts of cancer echoing in my head, and the bond continued to grow stronger. We had taken a journey together, and that journey had changed us forever, individually and as a team.

In November 2002, Bullet developed a cough that sounded just like a cat with fur balls. Being an experienced cat owner, I was so sure of my "diagnosis" that I gave him a hairball remedy for two days. But the cough persisted and off we went to the clinic.

Tests revealed that Bullet was in heart failure and was coughing because his lungs were filled with fluid. The diagnoses were dilated cardiomyopathy and atrial fibrillation. These maladies might or might not have been caused by doxorubicin, one of the chemotherapy agents in Bullet's protocol. Doxorubicin can cause cardiomyopathy, but generally it doesn't take two years for the damage to become apparent.

I felt that this was an extremely unfair turn of events. Wasn't it enough that my sweet boy had endured cancer and chemotherapy? Then it dawned on me that just because Bullet beat cancer, that didn't mean he would live forever. He would eventually die from something. This was such a simple concept, but it took me by surprise.

The veterinarians said that if we could get the fluid out of Bullet's lungs and control his heart conditions with medicine, he might survive another six months to a year ... or he could die suddenly at any time and I should be prepared for this eventuality. The medications did clear his lungs of fluid. He was given the same meds that are given to humans with these conditions, just as the chemotherapy agents used to fight canine cancer are pretty much the same as those that treat human cancer.

However, after considerable down-dosing, we found that Bullet could not tolerate digoxin, the one medication that could have reversed atrial fibrillation and allowed a normal heartbeat.

I was told many times by many veterinarians over the following two years that Bullet could die at any moment, without warning. I knew it was true, but Bullet and I agreed not to dwell on it. Over the next two years, I marveled at Bullet's strength as he just kept plodding along, brushing off all of the veterinarians' dismal doomsday predictions.

In April 2003, Bullet had a second left-sided heart failure, with the same coughing symptoms as the first. Dr. Hoskins consulted with a telemedicine service called Cardiopet. A cardiologist at the Advanced Veterinary Care Center in Newburgh, NY, evaluated Bullet's condition. We adjusted Bullet's medications and, once again, his lungs cleared.

In May 2003, Bullet and I participated in "Dogswalk Against Cancer," an event sponsored by the American Cancer Society. Part of the funds raised were granted to the Cornell University College of Veterinary Medicine for cancer research. Bullet completed the mile-and-a-half walk in good form.

In August 2003, we visited Margot and Dick Basile, dear friends and proprietors of the China Clipper, a B&B on Cape Cod. Margot and Dick were dog lovers par excellence. Complete and proper dog care was the top priority in the Basile household. When I awoke on the second day at the China Clipper, Bullet's neck and throat region became so full that he had no neck to speak of. I felt his lymph nodes, with trepidation, but they were not enlarged. I hoped that an increase in his furosemide dose would reduce the edema overnight, as it had in the past.

When I awoke the next morning, Bullet was lying on his side with absolutely no interest in getting up. His belly had become distended and hard overnight, and I knew that we were in very serious trouble. The Basiles' veterinarian made a house call to examine Bullet. After a short examination, she directed me to get him to a clinic posthaste—a clinic that had an ultrasound unit in-house. Of course, this was a Saturday afternoon. I knew that finding such a facility would be difficult.

That morning involved a frenzy of phone calls to local veterinary clinics, Dr. Porzio in Canada, Dr. Hoskins in New York, and old acquaintances at nearby Tufts Vet School. Tracy and I packed up in no time flat and piled into my car, along with Bullet, Toshi, and Kai. During the two-hour white-knuckle drive to the twenty-four-hour emergency clinic at Tufts Vet School in North Grafton, MA, Bullet's condition worsened. I was racing the clock, balancing my need to get to the clinic in time to save Bullet against getting there safely and without any police involvement.

Bullet stayed overnight at the hospital, and Tracy, Toshi, Kai, and I found a nearby motel that allowed dogs. It was congestive heart failure again, but this time both sides of his heart were in failure. Bullet's condition improved marginally overnight, with a nitroglycerine patch on his ear, an injection of furosemide, fluids, and constant monitoring. In the morning, I signed him out "against veterinarian's advice" to move him to a clinic near home.

After another two-hour white-knuckle car ride with two humans and three dogs, we arrived at the twenty-four-hour emergency animal hospital in Katonah-Bedford, NY. I called the clinic when we were ten minutes away and, at our arrival, two staff workers were waiting for us in the parking lot with a gurney, ready to transport Bullet into the hospital.

There were diagnostic tests and again revisions in Bullet's cardiac medications. He now had to be given a much higher dose of furosemide to prevent his lungs from filling up with fluid, and this meant lots of drinking and lots of peeing. It also meant that we were approaching the maximum dosage of furosemide. We would soon reach the place where we could no longer increase his dosage to fight congestive heart failure.

Bullet did recover once again but was not his old spunky self. Dr. Porzio suggested a cardiac medication for dogs not yet approved for use in the United States.. Through the Internet, I was able to correspond with several people whose dogs had been given this medication in clinical trials and survived several additional years with good quality of life.

Bullet was not eligible to participate in an ongoing clinical trial for this medication because of his history of lymphoma. However, the veterinary cardiologist who gave me this news also explained how to go about getting the drug for Bullet. After finding a pharmacist in Great Britain who was willing to export Vetmedin® (pimobendan), I arranged for the FDA to fax the necessary forms to Dr. Hoskins. A week after he filed these, we had FDA permission to import this wonder drug, which is now FDA approved and readily available in the United States.

Very soon after beginning daily doses of this medication, Bullet's energy level and quality of life improved greatly. He regained his spunk and his "growly bear" -ness. My gleeful reaction when he growled and chewed on a friend's hand may have seemed strange to some, but to me these were signs that Bullet was himself again.

On March 15, 2004, Bullet turned thirteen years old. As always, passersby stopped us on every outing with questions about Bullet, stories about other Siberians, and great praise for his beauty and grace.

At this time, Bullet was in good form, with excellent quality of life. It seemed we had all of his issues under control. There were episodes of congestive heart failure now and again—five in all—but these were resolved by adjusting his medication or giving a furosemide injection. Sometimes I thought we could go on like this indefinitely, with his cancer and heart conditions holding steady.

Along with the increased dosage of furosemide came increased drinking and increased urination. I looked for a doggie diaper. I found one, but would require pulling Bullet's great big furry tail through a small hole. I didn't have to attempt this to know that it was not going to work for us.

I created a simple diaper holder on my sewing machine, into which I could place a baby diaper swaddle/snuggle insert. The diaper holder worked quite well, but what didn't occur to me until it was too late was that with a diaper on, Bullet wasn't able to clean himself, and the area remained constantly wet.

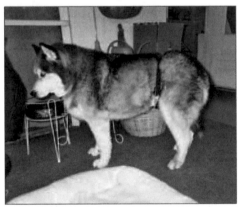

In the summer of 2004 there was a heat wave in New York. Bullet was indoors (and diapered) all of the time except for quick trips outdoors to relieve himself. He developed a urinary tract infection, which was cleared up by antibiotics. After this, Bullet wore diapers only during certain parts of the day, giving him time to keep himself clean and air out.

In May 2004, I discovered a grape-sized tumor on Bullet's side. I immediately stopped feeding him oatmeal and reinstated most of his cancer supplements. A needle biopsy report said that the tumor was most likely malignant. The recommendation was to "remove with wide margins."

"How would you feel," I asked Dr. Hoskins, "about operating on a thirteen-year-old husky with lymphoma and heart disease?" He thought about it and said that he felt Bullet was strong enough to tolerate the surgery. I reached out to Bullet's cancer team members for advice. Unanimously, the consensus was to remove the tumor with wide margins. I scheduled surgery to occur just after the American Cancer Society's 2004 Dogswalk Against Cancer at Bear Mountain.

Bullet was selected as King of the Dogswalk. Coincidentally, the Queens of the Dogswalk were two cancer dogs whose owners and I had met online at the Delphi Forums Pet Cancer Support Group. In May 2004, Bullet, Suzi (Hanon), and Diamond Dreamer (Furstinger) were crowned and admired by all. The royal families then proudly led the procession of people and dogs around Bear Mountain Lake.

The following week, Dr. Hoskins called upon Bullet's cardiac team to recommend the anesthesia to be used during surgery. The surgery was performed by board-certified surgeon Dr. Martin DiAngelis, assisted by Dr. Hoskins.

The tumor was the size of a grape; the tissue removed was the size of a grapefruit. As always, Dr. Hoskins was respectful of my aversion to seeing bare skin on Bullet and was diligent about shaving no more fur than necessary.

Making the decision to have the surgery was easy. In my mind, there was no alternative. Bullet was moving slowly and showing signs of old age, but was still full of personality and enjoying life. When the biopsy report from this surgery described a highly aggressive nerve sheath cancer, it confirmed that aggressive removal had been the right course of action regardless of the outcome. Bullet tolerated the surgery but, not surprisingly for a fellow with cancer and heart disease at his advanced age, his recovery was slow.

In July 2004, the first edition of this book, *Help Your Dog Fight Cancer*, was published. Bullet continued to recover as the book continued to find its way to people who had dogs with cancer. Each order that came through brought sadness. But remembering how desperately I had wanted a book like this one four years earlier, each order also makes me glad that I had the book to offer.

By October 2004, Bullet was having difficulty walking. His rear legs were failing, and there was little we could do to help apart from surgery, which was out of the question. We went to Cape Cod for what would be our last visit to the Basiles and walked a bit on the beach in the rain. We didn't mind. At this point, Bullet's hind legs were weakening and worsening, so I purchased a wonderful custom-made cart for him from Eddie's Wheels, in Shelburne Falls, MA.

November 15, 2004, Bullet virtually stopped walking and then stopped eating. A blood test showed that he was in kidney failure and he was dehydrated. I wasn't willing to leave him at the hospital overnight where he might die without me. So an IV catheter was installed in his leg, and I set him up in my bedroom with IV fluids. I hoped as always for a recovery, but felt that Bullet might not have any more miracles left.

I prepared a new diet with a lower protein content for his kidneys, put it through a food processor, and added water until it had the consistency of a thick soup for force-feeding. Force-feeding is really just a matter of spooning food into a large tube and then slowly emptying it (by pressing on the plunger) into the patient's mouth. Bullet was very cooperative about smacking his lips and swallowing the food. I gave him water in the same manner.

On Thursday, November 18, after three days of IV fluids, a blood test showed that Bullet's kidneys had improved. An on-call veterinarian cautioned me not to be optimistic. This test was performed in-house, and the previous one at a laboratory. The apparent improvement could have been due simply to differing calibrations. He said, "You don't see kidney values like these in living dogs." He said it was time. I said that if his kidneys did not improve by Monday, I would take that step.

Dr. Hoskins called on the morning of November 20, to say that Bullet's blood test results from Friday showed significant improvement. He seemed hopeful that the Magic Bullet might have just one more magic trick left in his bag. Perhaps Bullet really could cheat death just one more time.

Ten minutes later, Bullet died in my arms. I began mouth-to-nose resuscitation, but after a minute I stopped. I said, *"Oh, no … wait a minute … maybe I shouldn't be doing this."* I looked down at his sweet face. He was so beautiful lying there as though asleep, so peaceful. It shocked and pained me when I realized that I was not going to try to resuscitate him. That I was not going to see him awaken. That he would never again look at me with those beautiful ice-blue eyes, not ever again. Our long, long journey had come to an end, and all I could think was, *"No, wait, please wait! I'm not finished taking care of you."*

The phone number for the Hartsdale Pet Cemetery and Crematory had been tacked to my bulletin board for four years. I had glanced at it hundreds of times, thinking with a smile, *"I don't need you yet."* Now I made the call, and within two hours a young man came to carry Bullet's body, gently and respectfully, from my house to the station wagon.

The cremation was three days later. My friend Lynn and I were ushered into a small room to say good-bye. Bullet was a bit cold to the touch, but otherwise he looked and felt just exactly as he did when I had last saw him. Lynn said it was amazing how beautiful he was, even in death. The following day, I returned to pick up the cremains.

The days that followed were difficult. I no longer had to take him outside every two hours. I was free to go on whole-day outings at will. The constant trips to the vet's office had stopped as had the dosings of medications and supplements. And yet, I would gladly, without hesitation, have given up all of these newfound freedoms for another decade or another minute with Bullet.

I missed his head on my arm in the car. I missed watching my fingers disappear as they stroked his luxurious, deep, soft fur. I missed his cold nose touching my face as a peck more than a kiss. I missed feeling my heart melt when I turned a corner or raised my head from my work to catch him watching me. I missed the stirring in my heart and the awe that Bullet brought me, comparable to standing at the edge of the Grand Canyon, and looking in amazement at what nature has made.

I missed the first eighteen months of Bullet's life, and I'm grateful that I was given the opportunity to keep him by my side during his twilight years. I'm glad that neither of the beasts—cancer nor heart disease—took him in the end.

This is the story of a very special dog, "The love of my life, the dog of my dreams." It's the story of a shelter dog once named Max who came to be known as Bullet, who earned the titles of Bully, Bullet Growly Bear, and King Bully, and who will be remembered with love as the Magic Bullet.

I'm forever grateful that such a remarkable creature graced my life for one shining moment that lasted twelve years, two months, and a day.

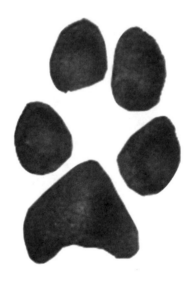

Appendices

Search the Internet

One of the best ways to gather current information is on the Internet. There is a wealth of information, but it's a double-edged sword. You will find the most up to date, current cutting edge information, but you will also find a lot of not so current, not so accurate information.

Explore web sites managed by veterinary schools (see Appendix). Other reliable resources on the net include web sites for any major veterinary specialty clinic, and veterinary organizations including www.vetcancersociety.org, www.avma.org and www.gcvs.com/oncology.

Open a search engine and start plugging in words. It might take you a while and several word combinations before you find what you're looking for—be patient. Use various combinations such as "chemotherapy dogs," "canine cancer," or "veterinary oncology," or the name of your dog's cancer followed by "canine," or "dogs," or "veterinary."

At each web site, you'll find links to other sites. Click on any links that pique your interest. Save good web sites as "bookmarks" or "favorites," or print out important pages. As you link from web site to web site, you will inevitably forget where you started.

Use a search engine to research medications and treatments, supplements, clinical trials and diets or for a particular type of canine cancer. If you hear of a supplement that might help your dog, open your search engine and type in its name to search for information about it.

The Internet can be a wonderful resource, but some advice you come across may not be appropriate for your dog. Some advice or claims may not be true or accurate. Check the source and validity of information that you find on the net before adding it to your treatment plan. Discuss it with your veterinarian and with the members of an online support group.

Join a Support Group!

Online support groups for people with cancer dogs are invaluable. We all get information from our veterinarians. It is important to also get information from other dog owners, who are not veterinarians, who have nothing to gain or lose because of the decisions we make, and who can relate to our experience as a dog owner who has a dog with cancer.

Participate if you choose to, or just read the questions, answers, and advice posted by others.

Pet Cancer Support (Search in Facebook for the group)

I joined this group a year after Bullet's diagnosis. I was shocked to find that there were so many others who were fiercely fighting to beat their dog's cancer.

In the Pet Cancer Support group, I found an active exchange of information about canine cancer as well as encouragement and compassion. Members are well versed about all aspects of canine cancer and will offer you all the support you will need. You may even make some lifelong friends in this group as I did.

Lymphoma Heart Dogs (Search in Facebook for this group)

Lymphoma Heart Dogs is specifically for owners of dogs with lymphoma. The group discusses information about medical and alternative treatments for lymphoma. The group offers loving support for the members to help each other through a very difficult time.

Bone Cancer Dogs (Search in Facebook for this group)

If you have a dog with osteosarcoma (bone cancer) it is very important to join this group. You will find people who know a great deal about all of the very difficult decisions you will have to make, and the pros and cons of each decision. The well-informed and dedicated members of this group have a personal understanding of the emotional journey involved in caring for a dog with osteosarcoma.

Vaccination Waiver

Date _____

Caretaker's Name _____

Address _____

Dog's Name _____ Birth Date _____

Sex _____ Breed _____

    I certify that I have examined the animal described. To the best of my knowledge and belief, the statements indicated below are true.

1. This dog to the best of my knowledge has been free from infectious, contagious and/or communicable disease for the past _____ days/months.
2. This dog is in good physical condition   YES   NO
3. The dog's caretaker states no known exposure to rabies or other communicable diseases within the past _____ days/months.
4. The county of residence is not under a rabies quarantine. YES NO
5. The caretaker states that the animal has not bitten anyone within the last 10 days. YES NO

_____ *I recommend that this animal be exempt from the requirement for rabies vaccination because the rabies vaccines, as instructed by the vaccine manufacturers, are for use in healthy animals only.*

_____ *The animal named above is not considered to be healthy because this animal is currently in treatment for this medical condition:* _____.

_____ *The animal named above has had an anaphylactic reaction to a prior rabies vaccination and further vaccination could result in serious illness or death.*

_____   _____   _____

Veterinarian's Signature   License Number   Date

Permission granted to print for personal use.

Early Warning Signs

SIGNS YOU CAN FEEL

- Abnormal Swellings that continue to grow in the skin, including enlarged lymph nodes (see illustrations)
- Abnormal Lumps in the mouth, mammary glands, testicles, abdomen or at vaccine sites
- Sores or Ulcers that do not heal in two weeks on the nose, ear tips and face, seen particularly on white cats and on the white underside skin of dogs such as Italian Grey Hounds, Whippets and Bulldogs

SIGNS YOU CAN SEE

- Sudden or Progressive Weight Loss: Use a baby scale to weigh cats and small dogs
- Pale Gums and Mucous Membranes: Yellow (jaundice) membranes; bruising; slow or inadequate refill
- Bad Breath: Halitosis or more than one loose tooth at same location
- Abdominal: Distended abdomen; fluid in the abdomen
- Skin: Small red spots or red discoloration of the skin; unexplained bleeding at any location, especially from body openings

SIGNS YOU CAN OBSERVE

- Decreased Appetite: Eating less than usual; walking away from bowl, refusing treats
- Reduced Activity: Lethargy; exercise intolerance; lameness; painful movement; painful joints; hesitation to exercise
- Abnormal Urination: Difficulty urinating; blood in the urine; excessive urine output; increased water drinking
- Abnormal Defecation: Loose stools; diarrhea; straining to defecate; constipation; blood or mucus in the stool
- Gastrointestinal: Difficulty eating; excessive salivation; spitting up food; vomiting food or bile
- Respiratory: Chronic sneezing; discharge from the eyes; unilateral nasal discharge; noisy breathing; trouble breathing; coughing; gagging
- Cardiovascular: Weakness; disorientation; dizziness, paralysis; pain; fainting; breathlessness; increased panting; anxiety

Ask your veterinarian to demonstrate the at home check-up.
Provided by Alice Villalobos, DVM

Chemotherapy Protocols

When chemotherapy is the treatment of choice, there may be a decision to be made about which protocol to use.

For dogs with osteosarcoma having chemotherapy, the protocol used is generally **single-agent carboplatin**, or **carboplatin alternating with adri-amycin**, for a total of 6 treatments, given three weeks apart.

Most of the dogs given chemotherapy protocols are the dogs with lymphoma. There are three main chemotherapy options for lymphoma.

▶   The Single-Agent Adriamycin protocol consists of five treatments with Adriamycin, given three weeks apart.

▶   The CCNU (or CeeNU) protocol uses a drug called Lomustine. It is given as a pill and can be given at home with visits to the clinic for blood tests every three to four weeks. This is a less expensive option. It is a good option for aggressive or fearful dogs, to avoid clinic visits. More often, this protocol is used as a rescue protocol, when a dog comes out of remission after a COP or CHOP protocol.

▶   A **COP** protocol uses the same drugs as the CHOP protocol below, but without Adriamycin. When a dog comes out of remission, then Adria is used for rescue.

▶   Most often, one of the **CHOP** protocols is used. These protocols have been found to be the most effective and provide the longest survival times. They include the following drugs:

C = Cyclophosphamide (Cytoxan)
H = Adriamycin (H for hydroxydaunorubicin)
O = Vincristine (O for Oncovin)
P = Prednisone

A CHOP protocol may also include L-Spar (Asparaginase) alone or with Vincristine for the first treatment. Including L-Spar as a first treatment is said not to improve the efficacy of the protocol.

The most popular and most often used CHOP protocol is the Modified Madison Wisconsin Protocol.

The Modified Madison-Wisconsin Protocol

Includes prednisone, not shown. Week 1 may or may not include L-Spar. Cytoxan may be intravenous at clinic or pills given at home.

Week	Drug	Date	Your Notes
1	Vincristine		
2	Cytoxan		
3	Vincristine		
4	Adriamycin		
Week off, no treatment			
6	Vincristine		
7	Cytoxan		
8	Vincristine		
9	Adriamycin		
Every other week from here on			
11	Vincristine		
13	Cytoxan		
15	Vincristine		
17	Adriamycin		
19	Vincristine		
21	Cytoxan		
23	Vincristine		
25	Adriamycin		
End of Protocol			

Permission granted to print for personal use.

The "Re-Modified" Modified Madison-Wisconsin Protocol

Since about 2014, some veterinary oncologists and veterinarians have been using variations (re-modified versions) of the Modified Madison-Wisconsin protocol. A very common variation is below. Cytoxan may be given in pill form rather than IV, and then the owner can receive the pills on weeks 5, 9 and 13 to give at home. In effect, the in-clinic treatments are reduced to every other week.

Week	Drug	Date	Your Notes
1	Vincristine		
2	Cytoxan		
3	Adriamycin		
Week off, no treatment			
5	Vincristine		
6	Cytoxan		
7	Adriamycin		
Week off, no treatment			
9	Vincristine		
10	Cytoxan		
11	Adriamycin		
Week off, no treatment			
13	Vincristine		
14	Cytoxan		
15	Adriamycin		
End of protocol			
*Some provide two more treatments with Adriamycin, 3 weeks apart			

Permission granted to print for personal use.

The MOPP Protocol

Day	Drug	Your Notes
0	Mustargen 3.0 mg/m2	
0	Vincristine .75 mg/m2	
0	Porcarbazine 50 mg/m2 x14 days	
0	Pred 30 mg/m2 x 14 days	
7	Mustargen 3.0 mg/m2	
7	Vincristine .75 mg/m2	
28	Mustargen 3.0 mg/m2	
28	Vincristine .75 mg/m2	
28	Porcarbazine 50 mg/m2 x14 days	
28	Pred 30 mg/m2 x 14 days	
35	Mustargen 3.0 mg/m2	
35	Vincristine .75 mg/m2	
	Repeat	

The Single-Agent Adriamycin Protocol

Week	Drug	Your Notes
0	Adriamycin	
3	Adriamycin	
6	Adriamycin	
9	Adriamycin	
12	Adriamycin	
End of Protocol - No more than five Adria treatments should be given		

Permission granted to print for personal use.

The CCNU Rescue Protocol

The CCNU, or CeeNU or Lomustine protocol, is given orally every three weeks and Prednisone every other day. Pills may be given by the owner at home. Periodic blood tests are needed before some treatments, to ensure the correct dosage.

A dog out of remission may be given prednisone alone to prolong survival time for a few months. CCNU may provide a few additional months. This protocol continues until it is no longer working.

This protocol is for:
▸ Dogs who have come out of remission from a CHOP protocol such as the Modified Madison/Wisconsin Protocol, given as a rescue protocol.
▸ Owners who cannot afford the CHOP protocol
▸ Dogs who are aggressive or fearful and dogs are not good candidates for weekly treatments at clinic, but can be pilled at home by owner.

The Modified CCNU Rescue Protocol

Recently popular, L-Spar is given with the first two CCNU treatments. CCNU treatments are given every three weeks for five treatments, or until the cancer progresses. "Until the cancer progresses" means until the dog's quality of life has declined and treatment is abandoned.

A small study of 31 dogs is published as "Combination Chemotherapy with L-Asparaginase, Lomustine, and Prednisone for Relapsed or Refractory Canine Lymphoma," in *Journal of Veterinary Internal Medicine*, Volume 21, Issue 1. In this study, survival times are no better than the original CCNU protocol, without L-Spar.

Carboplatin x 5

Generally used for osteosarcoma, after amputation. IV Carboplatin is given every three weeks for a total of five treatments. May be alternated with adriamycin (three treatments with each drug, total of 6 treatments).

Vinblastine x 8

Protocol is often used for mast cell cancer, or dogs with osteosarcoma after amputation, or other cancers. Vinblastine is given once a week for four treatments, and every other week for four more treatments.

Chemotherapy Drugs

Generic/brand Name	Cancer Types	Administration	Common Side Effects
asparaginase, Elspar L-Spar (*B)	LSA, Leukemia	IM; SubQ	Anaphylaxis, mild myelo, pancreatitis
bleomycin, Blenoxane®	Carcinomas, LSA, Leukemia	SubQ; IL	Mild myelo, Kidney, Liver
carboplatin, Paraplatin®	Osteosarcoma, Melanoma	IV infusion	Myelo, GI, allergy
chlorambucil, Leukeran®	LSA, Leukemia, STT, MCT	Oral	Moderate myelo
cyclophosphamide, Cytoxan® (*F)	LSA, Leukemia, STT, Mmc	Orally; IV	Severe myelo, GI, bleeding cystitis
cytarabine, Cytoxar-U®	Leukemia, LSA	IV	Myelo
dacarbazine, DTIC-Dome®	Relapsed LSA	IV	Severe vomiting; myelo
dactinomycin	LSA, rhabdomyosarcoma	IV	Myelo, GI
doxorubicin, Adriamycin® (*B)	LSA, Leukemia, OSA, HSA	IV infusion	Severe myelo, GI, anaphylaxis, cardiomyopathy
gemcitabine HCl Gemzar®	Pancreatic/Liver Carcinoma	IV	Myelo, vomiting, anaphylaxis
hydroxyurea, Hydrea®	Leukemia	Oral	GI, Mild myelo
lomustine CeeNU®, CCNU	Relapsed LSA, MCT	Oral	Myelo, GI, lungs
methotrexate, Trexsol®	LSA, Leukemia	IV	Moderate myelo, GI
mitoxantrone, Novantrone®	LSA, STT	IV infusion	Myelo, anaphylaxis, GI
mechlorethamine, Mustargen®	LSA	IV	Myelo, anaphylaxis, GI
paclitaxel, Taxol®, Paclical® Vet	MCT, Mammary, OSA	IV	Myelo, anaphylaxis, GI
piroxicam, Feldene®	TCC, CMM, Carcinomas	Oral	GI ulceration (an anti-inflammatory)
Prednisone	LSA, Leukemia, Insulinoma	Oral	Thirst, urination, panting, mild myelo
Procarbazine	LSA, brain/lung cancer	Oral	GI, Neuromuscular
vinblastine, Velban®	LSA, Leukemia, MCT, STT	IV infusion	Severe myelo, GI
vincristine, Oncovin®	LSA, Leukemia, MCT, STT	IV	Mild-moderate myelo, GI, Neurological
vinorelbine (*B)	MCT, lung cancer	IV	Myelo, GI, Neurological

Key to Abbreviations

After drug name: (*B)=pretreat with Benadryl; (*F) = pretreat with furosemide
Cancer Type: LSA=Lymphoma; CMM=Canine malignant melanoma;
TCC=Transitional cell carcinoma; STT–Soft tissue tumors. MCT=Mast cell tumor;
OSA=Osteosarcoma; HSA=Hemangiosarcoma; Mmc=Mammary (breast) cancer
Administration: SubQ=Subcutaneous injection; IV=Intravenous; IM=Intramuscular
injection; IL=Intralesional
Side Effects: Myelo=Myelosuppression/Bone marrow; GI=Gastrointestinal;
Anaphylaxis=Severe potentially fatal allergic reaction

Chemo Notes

▶ Every dog reacts differently to each chemo drug. Don't anticipate a crash just because of a drug's bad reputation. Don't be surprised if your dog has side effects from a drug that usually does not cause side effects.

▶ If your dog has side effect of vomiting after treatment, ask your veterinarian to pretreat with Benadryl and/or antiemetics such as Cerenia. Your vet can also prescribe pills to give your dog at home for a day after chemotherapy treatment.

▶ Most treatments take about 20 minutes. Infusions take up to 2 hours.

▶ Watch for extravasation! Examine injection sites closely and report sores or eruptions to your veterinarian immediately.

▶ Protocols should be altered to manage side effects. Dosages can be reduced and schedules can be extended as needed.

▶ Treatment is postponed for a week when the white blood cell count (WBC) is low. Neutrophils (polys, absolute polys or ANC [absolute neutrophil count]) will also be low.

▶ Don't panic if treatment is postponed! This is very common. The WBC usually recovers within one week.

▶ Watch for neuropathy. If your dog is limping or knuckling, or reluctant to be active, tell your veterinarian.

▶ If your dog cannot tolerate chemotherapy, be prepared to switch to a rescue protocol or palliative care.

Data in Chemotherapy Drugs chart collected from Small Animal Clinical Oncology (W.B. Saunders Co), Manual of Small Animal Internal Medicine (Mosby), Veterinary Oncology Secrets (Hanley & Belfus, Inc.) and drug monographs as well as suggestions provided by several veterinary oncologists.

Schools of Veterinary Medicine

School	Phone
Auburn University	334-844-2685
University of California-Davis	530-752-1393 / 0186
Colorado State University	970-297-4195
Cornell University	607 253-3060
University of Florida	352-392-4700
University of Georgia	706-542-3461
University of Illinois-Urbana	217-333-5300
Iowa State University	515-294-4900
Kansas State University	785-532-5690
Louisiana State University	225-578-9600
Michigan State University	517-353-4523 / 5420
University of Minnesota	612-625-1919
Mississippi State University	662-325-1351 / 3432
University of Missouri	573-882-7821 / 4589
North Carolina State University	919-513-6690
Ohio State University	614-293-7517
Oklahoma State University	405-744-6648
Oregon State University	541-737-2858
University of Pennsylvania	215-898-4680 / 4685
Purdue University	765-494-1107
University of Tennessee	865-974-8387
Texas A&M University	979-845-2351
Tufts University	508-839-5395
Tuskegee University	334-727-8436
Virginia-Maryland Reg CVM	540-231-4621
Washington State University	509-335-0711
University of Wisconsin-Madison	608-263-7600

Permission granted to print for personal use.

Website
http://www.vetmed.auburn.edu/animal-owners/bailey/specialties-and-services/oncology/
http://www.vetmed.ucdavis.edu/vmth/small_animal/oncology/index.cfm
www.csuanimalcancercenter.org
http://www.vet.cornell.edu/hospital/Services/Companion/Oncology/
http://smallanimal.vethospital.ufl.edu/clinical-services/oncology/
http://www.vet.uga.edu/hospital/services/oncology_sa
http://vetmed.illinois.edu/vth/dogs_cats_services.html
http://vetmed.iastate.edu/vmc/small-animal/medical-services/oncology-service
http://www.vet.k-state.edu/vhc/services/small/oncology/
http://www1.vetmed.lsu.edu/VTHC/Shared%20Services/Oncology/item26469.html
http://cvm.msu.edu/hospital/services/oncology-service
http://www.cvm.umn.edu/vmc/specialties/oncology/index.htm
http://cvm.msstate.edu/index.php/animal-health-center/companion-animals/
http://vmth.missouri.edu/oncology.htm
http://www.cvm.ncsu.edu/vhc/tc/clinical_services/onco/index.html
http://vet.osu.edu/vmc/companion/our-services/oncology-and-hematology
http://cvhs.okstate.edu/veterinary-teaching-hospital/services
http://vetmed.oregonstate.edu/hospital/oncology
http://www.vet.upenn.edu/veterinary-hospitals/ryan-veterinary-hospitalcancer-care/
http://www.vet.purdue.edu/vth/small-animal/oncology.php
https://vetmed.tennessee.edu/vmc/SmallAnimalHospital/Oncology/Pages/
http://vethospital.tamu.edu/small-animal-hospital/oncology
http://vet.tufts.edu/fhsa/veterinary_specialties/oncology.html
www.tuskegee.edu/academics/colleges/cvmnah/school_of_veterinary_medicine.aspx
http://www.vetmed.vt.edu/vth/oncology.asp
http://vth.vetmed.wsu.edu/specialties/oncology/information-for-owners/
http://uwveterinarycare.wisc.edu/small-animal/cats-and-dogs/oncology/

Permission granted to print for personal use.

Quality of Life Scale

The HHHHHMM Quality of Life scale will help you evaluate your dog's quality of life during pawspice.

For each heading below, circle a score. Zero is the worst and 10 is the best. A total score above 35 shows an acceptable Quality of Life for dogs to remain in pawspice care.

HURT 0 1 2 3 4 5 6 7 8 9 10

What is your pet's pain level? Is your pet's pain successfully managed with pain medications that provide comfort? Is breathing difficult? Is Oxygen necessary? If your pet is desperate for breath, this takes all priority and pawspice should end.

HUNGER 0 1 2 3 4 5 6 7 8 9 10

Does hand-feeding help maintain weight? Does your pet require a feeding tube?

HYDRATION 0 1 2 3 4 5 6 7 8 9 10

For pets not drinking enough water, provide sub cutaneous fluids once or twice daily, to supplement fluid intake.

HYGIENE 0 1 2 3 4 5 6 7 8 9 10

Your pet should be brushed and cleaned, particularly after eliminations. Avoid pressure sores by using soft bedding. Keep all wounds clean on a daily basis.

Permission granted to print this page for personal use.

HAPPINESS **0 1 2 3 4 5 6 7 8 9 10**

> *Does your dog express joy and interest? Is he responsive to things around him (family, toys, etc)? Is he depressed, lonely, anxious, bored or afraid? Put his bed in family activity areas so he won't feel isolated.*

MOBILITY **0 1 2 3 4 5 6 7 8 9 10**

> *** Score each question below 0=No, 10=Yes. Add up and divide by 5.*
> *Can your pet get up without assistance? __*
> *Does he feel like going for a walk? __*
> *Is he depressed? __*
> *Does he need human or mechanical help, or a cart? __*
> *Is your pet trembling, having seizures or stumbling? __*

MORE GOOD DAYS THAN BAD **0 1 2 3 4 5 6 7 8 9 10**

> *Do bad days outnumber good days? If so, quality of life might be too compromised to continue life. When a healthy human-animal bond is no longer possible, the caregiver must be made aware that the end is near. The final decision must be made if a pet is suffering so that death can come peacefully and painlessly.*

TOTAL SCORE: _____

Created by Dr. Alice Villalobos, who is available for consults. Schedule a consult online at www.Pawspice.com.
The HHHHHMM QoL Scale was originally published in "Canine and Feline Geriatric Oncology: Honoring the Human-Animal Bond," by Alice Villalobos, DVM, DPNAP, with Laurie Kaplan (Wiley-Blackwell, 2007) Reprinted with permission from Wiley-Blackwell.

Permission granted to print this page for personal use.

Reading List

Cancer-Specific Books

Advances in Veterinary Oncology, An Issue of Veterinary Clinics of North America: Small Animal Practice, by Annette N. Smith.

Cancer And Your Pet: The Complete Guide to the Latest Research, Treatments, and Options, by Debra Eldredge, DVM and Margaret H. Bonham.

Canine and Feline Geriatric Oncology: Honoring the Human-Animal Bond, by Alice Villalobos, DVM.

Dog Cancer: The Holistic Answer: A Step by Step Guide, by Dr. Steven Eisen.

Merck/Merial Manual for Pet Health (home edition).

Pets Living With Cancer: A Pet Owner's Resource, by Robin Downing, DVM.

The Dog Cancer Survival Guide: Full Spectrum Treatments to Optimize Your Dog's Life Quality and Longevity, by Demian Dressler, DVM and Susan Ettinger, DVM.

The Natural Vet's Guide to Preventing and Treating Cancer in Dogs, by Shawn Messonnier, DVM.

Veterinary Oncology Secrets, by Robert C. Rosenthal, DVM, PhD.

Why is Cancer Killing Our Pets?, by Deborah Straw.

Withrow and MacEwen's Small Animal Clinical Oncology, by Stephen J. Withrow DVM DACVS DACVIM and David M. Vail DVM DACVIM.

Essential Books for Any Dog Lover

Dr. Pitcairn's Complete Guide to Natural Health for Dogs & Cats, by Richard H. Pitcairn, DVM and Susan Hubble Pitcairn.

Kindred Spirits: How the Remarkable Bond Between Humans and Animals Can Change the Way We Live, by Allen M. Schoen, M.S. DVM.

Natural Health Bible for Dogs & Cats: Your A-Z Guide to Over 200 Conditions, Herbs, Vitamins, and Supplements, by Shawn Messonnier DVM.

Speaking for Spot: Be the Advocate Your Dog Needs to Live a Happy, Healthy, Longer Life, by Nancy Kay, DVM.

The Naturally Clean Home: 101 Safe and Easy Herbal Formulas for Non-Toxic Cleansers, by Karyn Siegel- Maier.

Inspirational Stories About Dogs with Cancer

42 Rules to Fight Dog Cancer: Real Stories and Practical Approaches to Dealing with Dog Cancer by Aimee Quemuel.

Grizz's Story A Greater Courage, by Jo Helms.

Sparky Fights Back : A Little Dog's Big Battle Against Cancer, by Josee Clerens, John Clifton.

Without Regret: A Handbook for Owners of Canine Amputees, by Susan Neal.

Index

Stories about dogs

31901059329633